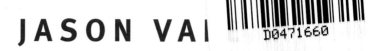

JASON VAI

the
Juice master
turbo-charge your life
in **14 days**

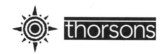

thorsons

By the same author:

The Juice Master's Slim 4 Life
The Juice Master's Ultimate Fast Food
Chocolate Busters

Thorsons
An Imprint of HarperCollins*Publishers*
77–85 Fulham Palace Road
Hammersmith, London W6 8JB

The website address is:
www.thorsonselement.com

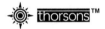 ™

and *Thorsons* are trademarks of
HarperCollins*Publishers* Limited

Published by Thorsons 2005

10 9

A catalogue record for this book
is available from the British Library

ISBN-13 978-0-00-719422-3
ISBN-10 0-00-719422-6

Printed and bound in Great Britain by
Martins the Printers Ltd, Berwick upon Tweed

Contents

Turbo-charge Changed My Life!

When I first wrote this book I was hoping that it would successfully inspire people to much better health and an improved lifestyle. However, I had no idea just how much difference it would make to so many people. I now receive many hundreds of emails and letters every week from people all over the world who have read the book, completed the programme and made unbelievable changes to their body shape, health and life.

Here are just a few *genuine* letters from the ever growing postbag – I hope, like the book itself, that they inspire you to an incredible life change.

'Just had to share my delight with you on completion of the 14-day Turbo-charge programme. I have lost 18lbs in 14 days! Truly amazing as I have tried them all before and never had such startling results with such ease and enjoyment. My husband looks and feels 10 years younger and is spreading the word to his "food police" mates. I overheard him explaining to one that "It isn't a diet, it's a permanent change of lifestyle."' **Alison**

'Four weeks ago I started the "Turbo-charge Your Life" programme, and now when I try to eat a fast-food burger I feel physically ill! I've lost weight, I look great, I feel great, and I'm bursting with energy for the first time in 15 years. I've never been happier. Thank you, Jason. For the paltry price of a juicer and your book, my life has changed completely. Best regards.' **Tony**

'Hi Jason, would just like to say thank you so much! I'm 15 and have been overweight all my life, constantly trying to slim down – that was until my mum bought your book, which I read. I've lost a stone (14lbs) and the weight just keeps going. I've never been happier or felt better. Thank you!' **Jenny**

THIS BOOK WORKS. READ IT – DO THE PROGRAMME – CHANGE YOUR LIFE IN JUST 14 DAYS

Take the Turbo-charge Challenge

FREE PLACE on Jason Vale's Mind and Body Detox retreat for the person who makes the biggest change on the Turbo-charge programme – see **www.thejuicemaster.com** for competition details or call 0044 (0) 8451 30 28 29.

Introduction

14 Days Guaranteed to Turbo-charge
Your Life for Ever

Let me make something very clear from the start: this book has been designed not simply to give you a kick up the backside on the health, fitness and life front, but to literally send a rocket booster up there!

It doesn't matter who you are, how many 'self-help' books you've read, how many seminars you've been to, how many times you've been on a diet or started an exercise programme in the past. It doesn't matter how much you may think you 'know it all' when it comes to this subject – the fact is we could all do with a bit of inspirational hard talking to move us from simply *thinking* about making a change 'one day' to actually getting off our backsides and just doing it.

The information in this book will not only help you to do just that, but *much* more importantly, it will explain exactly what is needed, on both a mental and physical level, to make the change stick for good. The last thing you want is what usually happens with virtually every health/fitness/diet/programme – you get all motivated, stick to it for a while, start looking and feeling good only to find yourself back where you started a few months down the line.

So many of us are good at the start. We are excited and have all the right intentions. But a massive 95 per cent of the time we revert back to our old ways and spend every weekend telling ourselves (and the world) that all will change again on … *Monday!*

My aim is simple: to supply you with the *correct* motivational, nutritional and fitness information to inspire you to complete the unique and highly effective 14-day Turbo-charge Your Life programme. I will also show you how to tap into the right psychology on a *regular* basis to enable you to create an amazing, compelling life where you truly live as opposed to 'survive'.

FAT Chance

I know that weight loss in particular is a huge issue for many people (pardon the pun), as indeed it was for myself for many years. This is hardly surprising as we are now in the unenviable position of holding the title of **'The Fattest Nation in Europe'** (and as you've no doubt seen that's up against some pretty big competition!). A massive three-quarters of the population of the UK are now classed as overweight or obese and children as young as 5 are now getting heart disease and 'early onset' diabetes. You cannot pick up a magazine or newspaper without mention of 'The Obese Time Bomb' waiting to explode. This is why I want to get something very clear from the start:

I can guarantee that you will lose 8–14 lb on the 14-day Turbo-charge Your Life programme.

That's if you need to lose weight clearly!

The weight loss I'm talking about here is in just the first 14 days, but as this programme will turbo-charge you for life, you will soon find you reach your ideal weight and body shape. What's even better is that the programme has also been designed to improve the skin, add body and shine to your hair, increase your energy levels and, more importantly, change the way you feel about food and exercise for ever.

The Turbo-charge Your Life programme is much, much more than a simple 'lose a few pounds' programme. In fact, not everyone follows the programme to lose weight. Many people simply want to feel light, to experience amazing health and tap into a level of raw energy they haven't had since they were children. Many people, especially men, also want to *increase* their weight by building muscle, which is why I want to make my second point very clear:

This programme is *not* just for overweight people.

Far from it. It has been designed for *everyone* who finds it hard either to kick-start or continue with a healthy, balanced eating and exercise programme. It's designed for all those who are fully aware of what they should eat for better health and why they should exercise more, but for some reason just cannot tap into the right frame of mind to get themselves to take action on a *consistent* basis. It's designed for those who have started many programmes in the past but never quite achieved their health and body potential. This unique programme is also designed for all those who not only want to improve their health, but also need the ultimate kick up the backside.

However, long before we get into the programme which will, without question, change your life, you have do the very thing that will make following the programme one of the most easy and enjoyable experiences you have ever had, and that is you must …

Read the Book!

We are living in an extremely bizarre time when it comes to health, exercise, meal preparation and dieting in general. As a nation we now have more cooking shows, more celebrity chefs and we buy more cookery books than any other country in Europe. However, we also buy more takeaways than any other country in Europe. In fact **the British spend £7,000 a minute on ready meals; that's three times more than any other country in Europe**. The projection is that we will be spending £5 billion on ready meals by 2007.

We also have more 'slimming' clubs, more health and exercise books and more celebrity 'get slim and fit' DVDs than any other country in Europe, yet we are also the fattest and most unhealthy country anywhere in Europe.

Why?

Because although we are good at buying the books, it appears we haven't actually mastered the art of reading them! Sure, we're good at flicking through them, but rarely, if ever, do we read the whole book and get around to acting on any of the information.

Virtually everyone I know has Jamie, Delia and Nigella in their kitchen, but I'll be damned if I've ever seen them cooking a recipe from any of them. These celeb cookery books have become the food equivalent of *Hello!* or *OK!* magazine – great for good food voyeurs, but unfortunately that's where it usually ends.

In the real world, most people have all the right intentions, but the reality remains the same. Most of us either grab a takeaway, tuck into a sandwich and crisps or shove a ready meal in the oven, believing *we've* made dinner! It appears that Jamie, Nigella and co aren't in the kitchen to help us prepare wonderful, wholesome food every night, but more as the ultimate kitchen fashion accessory.

In fact, I believe a big, glossy Jamie Oliver or a sultry Nigella book is now even more important to kitchen aesthetics than the Smeg hob itself. Gleaming state-of-the-art cookers remain gleaming, not because we are such super cleaners, but because we rarely actually turn them on.

At the same time, virtually every house I go into has some sort of self-help, diet or exercise book on the shelves, and yet the people who bought them are eating rubbish, watching hours of TV and complaining about their size, shape or lives in general. It was estimated that at the height of Atkins mania, 20 million people in the UK, Europe and the US were on the diet. However, what this figure actually meant was that 20 million people bought the book, but that doesn't mean Jack. Just because 20 million people had a copy doesn't mean for one second they actually read the book.

We need to remember that at *exactly* the same time Atkins made number one on the *New York Times* bestsellers list it was announced that for the first time in history over 60 per cent of the US population were considered overweight, obese or morbidly obese. Perhaps people weren't so much reading the books as eating them! Even the late Dr Atkins himself may have been guilty of this as, according to a popular UK newspaper, at the time of his death he weighed in at a whopping 250lbs.

Buying the book isn't enough – you have to read it!

I will tell you now that the information in this book *will* work. It *will* change the way you look at health and exercise. Without question, it will not just give you a good kick-start but will turbo-charge every single aspect of your life. I would even go as far as to say it would be impossible to read this book and not be moved in some way to change your eating and exercise habits and so, in turn, your life. As completely alien as it may seem at this stage, by the time you finish the book you will actually look forward to daily exercise, you will love the process of eating well and you will know exactly what is needed if you want to turbo-charge any aspect of your life. But, let me make this point crystal clear, if you simply flick through the book, use it as a place mat or leave it on your shelf, then it's got about as much chance of weaving its magic as George W Bush has of winning the Nobel Peace Prize!

Ninety-five per cent of self-help books remain unread on people's shelves.

Many people seem to think that by merely buying a book like this, they've done enough. You know what I mean. You feel good about the fact you're at least taking steps towards a better body and life. Then you get home, have a quick flick, put it down and say, 'I'll just do this and then I'll read it.' Next thing you know, there are more things to do and now the book's getting in the way. You then move it to one side and say, 'Tomorrow – I'll read it tomorrow!' But once again you get caught up with the 'more important' things, and before you know what's happened the book has found its way into a box or onto the bookshelf, never to see the light of day again. But at least you felt you were doing good for a moment – the moment you bought it.

It's similar to all those people who feel good about joining a gym, but simply joining a gym will not get you fit – YOU HAVE TO GO! Equally, buying this book will be about as much use as a pork pie at a Jewish wedding unless you actually read it *and* act on the information.

As you have probably gathered, I'm pretty keen to get this point across and I am not averse to repeating myself to make myself heard. The reason I do this is not to treat my readers as if they're a few biscuits short of the full packet, but because the more you hear something, the more it goes into both your conscious and subconscious mind.

To make absolutely certain that you know just how important I regard my first point, and with the danger of repeating myself again, I have dedicated a whole page to hammer the point home:

READ THE BOOK

read the book read the book read the book read the book read the book read the book read the book

read the book *read the book* read the book *read the book*

read the book read the book *read the book* read the book

read the book **read the book** read the book

read the book read the book

read the book *read the book* read the book

read the book read the book read the book read the book read the book read the book read the book

READ THE BOOK

read the book read the book read the book read the book read the book read the book read the book

read the book read the book *read the book* read the book

read the book read the book

read the book **read the book** *read the book*

read the book read the book read the book read the book read the book

read the book read the book read the book read the book read the book read the book read the book

read the book read the book *read the book* read the book

read the book read the book read the book read the book read the book read the book read the book

READ THE BOOK

Glad that's clear!

Don't just read the book, but read it in the order it was intended to be read, from start to finish. Being about the most impatient person I know, I'm fully aware that despite my massive 'READ THE BOOK' message, you may still be tempted to go straight to the 14-day Turbo-charge Your Life plan and just get on with it. But please, please, please don't. I will tell you now that if you do that, if you ignore my first piece of advice, the programme could well feel like just another diet/detox and exercise plan, and ultimately you will fail. Before you launch yourself into this life-changing programme, you *must* be mentally prepared *first* – it's the *mental* preparation that makes the difference between turbo-charging then crashing and turbo-charging, remaining up there and achieving the body, health and lifestyle you crave. If you're not dedicated enough to simply read the book, you've also got to ask yourself what possible hope you have of being committed to the programme itself.

Fortunately, as you can probably tell, I write the way I speak, so you will find you whiz through this book in no time at all. For those people who have never sampled my books before, you will see as we go on that I'm not here to win any literature awards. I'm here simply to help you get the results you're looking for. And if that means repeating certain points 20 times over, SHOUTING MY POINT, mildly swearing (at times) or being pretty blunt, then so be it. I don't expect you to agree with everything I write, or even to like my style all of the time, but as long as you use your intelligence, taking what makes sense to *you* and dumping what doesn't, you'll find your life will excel. Sometimes you can read just one line of a book and it triggers something that changes you for ever. All I ask is for you to be open-minded throughout.

So if you're ready to begin a journey that will turbo-charge every single aspect of your life, let's begin …

RULES OF THE BOOK

1. Read Chapters 1 to 8 in order. **2. Read at least one chapter of the book every day to keep your momentum.**

3. Follow the 14-day programme to the letter. rules of the book

1. READ CHAPTERS 1 TO 8 IN ORDER.

2. Read at least one chapter of the book every day to keep your momentum.

3. Follow the 14-day programme to the letter.

rules of the book *1. Read Chapters*

1 to 8 in order. **2. READ AT LEAST ONE CHAPTER OF THE BOOK EVERY DAY TO KEEP YOUR MOMENTUM.**

3. Follow the 14-day programme to the letter. *rules of the book*

1. Read Chapters 1 to 8 in order.

2. Read at least one chapter of the book every day to keep your momentum. 3. Follow the 14-day programme to the letter.

rules of the book **1. READ CHAPTERS 1 TO 8 IN ORDER.** 2. Read at least one chapter of the book every day to keep your momentum. *3. Follow the 14-day programme to the letter.* **rules of the book**

Quote of the Decade

Every now and then you hear just one sentence that not only warms your heart but also has the power to completely change the way you view your world, and in some cases to completely change your life. The following short story should help you change the way you look at your body and what you put into it.

An 87-year-old man was interviewed for a local Irish television station in the 1970s. He had been living on the streets for many years, but despite having no home or job he looked not just OK, but super well and healthy. He was also incredibly happy and explained that living on the street was a lifestyle choice as he loved being a 'free spirit'. When asked what his secret was he replied, 'It's simple. I don't eat any junk food.'

Now clearly this man didn't have a chance to cook, but he was incredibly fussy about what he put into his body and made sure he got plenty of good, nutrient-packed food every day. It turned out that he would go to the markets at the end of the day and get a couple of bags of fresh fruit, vegetables and nuts. He also got friendly with some restaurant owners who would, every now and then, rustle him up some wholesome cooked food.

When the interviewer asked him why he insisted on never eating junk food, he replied with a sentence that has to be one of the most profound ever aired, and you may need to read it twice, or at least think about it for a few seconds to fully understand it. His exact words were:

" The reason why I **don't eat junk food** is because if I don't look after my body, **I'll have nowhere to live.** "

And how true is that for all of us? If we don't look after our body we really will have nowhere to live. We may have somewhere to *survive*, but rarely will we experience the mental and physical vibrancy that will enable us to truly excel in *every* area of our life; rarely will we feel the power of what it's like to live every day in a powerful, light, slim, trim, energy-driven body.

It's No Good Being the Richest Person in the Graveyard!

I know that may sound over-dramatic, but as a former fat, chain-smoking heavy drinker, who grew up in a very rough part of London, experience has taught me a valuable lesson. There's a world of difference between just 'getting through' life, surviving from day to day, and having the raw energy to truly suck the juice out of each and every day.

The old man who lived on the streets would be seen by many as poor. But mentally and physically he was far wealthier than most people. He may not have had financial wealth, but he was truly *content* with his life – something most people never achieve – and his health bank account was well and truly in the black, something most people only dream of.

Now at this stage I already know you are financially much, much better off than that man, but no matter how much money you have, unless you are physically and mentally wealthy – you are poor. Unless you wake up looking forward to the adventures that the day may bring – you are poor. Unless you love your body and have the raw energy to play and excel every day – you are poor. Unless you have the energy to manifest your dreams – you are poor. If you 'can't be bothered' – you are poor. If you spend your life working from morning till night in a job you hate and are exhausted at the end of each day – you are poor.

Amazing health, like true love and affection, is about the only thing you cannot buy or cheat at – you can only *do* health.

No matter how much money you spend on liposuction, external creams, magic potions, botox or plastic surgery, the fact remains that you cannot buy mental and physical vibrancy – you can only earn it.

Digging Your Grave with Your Teeth

Your body is without question the single most important thing you will ever have the good fortune to use while you're on this planet, and yet most people are digging their own graves with their teeth. Everything we eat and drink; the way we move, or *don't* move our bodies; the environment we live in and how we think all affect our entire biochemistry and every single aspect of our lives. Your life and how you feel on a daily basis is a direct reflection of your internal and external health. When your body feels good, you feel good, and when you feel good, you are more productive, content and happy in every single area of your life.

The fact is, like that wise old man said, if you don't look after your body, you really will have nowhere to live. That is why most of this book focuses on what you put into your mouth and how you move your body, as without the right fuel for your body and mind it's almost impossible to turbo-charge your life and live your dreams.

Equally, if you don't look after your *mental* health – the thoughts you have daily; the way you see the world – you will also have nowhere to truly live.

Our thinking determines everything we do: our food choices; what we drink; whether we exercise; our work; how productive we are; how much love we give and what we strive for in life.

The way we think can also generate incredible stress, which can be more damaging to physical health than the worst foods and drinks on the planet. This is why as well as focusing on the most amazing super-fuel for the body, which will power you to amazing physical health, I will also be concentrating on changing the way you *think* about food, exercise and life in general.

Unless you change the way you think, everything remains the same.

No More *Excuses!*

There is nothing stopping anyone from getting the body and energy levels they crave – except excuses. You have clearly picked up this book because you are not 100 per cent happy on the health, fitness and body front. The reality is that there is nothing stopping you from taking the steps *right now* **that will get you the body and energy levels you crave. Nothing that is except ... excuses!**

If you think about it, most diets/programmes designed for weight loss and health do actually work, on a physical level at least. If you eat less and exercise more, the end result is usually weight loss – hardly rocket science! Equally, for those looking to gain weight, this can be achieved by eating more of the right muscle-building foods and doing a regular weight-lifting programme. And if you are the correct weight but find your energy levels on the floor, then you know that eating and drinking more 'live energy' foods and drinks and doing plenty of exercise will make you feel more energetic – once again, a degree in common sense is not required.

It's not so much that people don't know what to do to get a lean and healthy body and mind. Due purely to fear, they come up with a million excuses as to why they can't do it at this time. And boy will people make excuse after excuse. I call it 'the but syndrome'. '*But* I can't because ... *I'm too old.' 'But* I can't because … *I don't have the time.' 'But* I can't because … *blah, blah, blah.'* People who suffer from the but syndrome usually end up with a very big one – BUTT that is! Whatever 'but because' excuses you have, not only do they prevent you from getting what you really want, but I can guarantee they are a load of old rubbish. When looked at, none of these excuses hold any water at all.

The only way to stop having a big butt is to stop having a big 'but'!

Please do not make the mistake of looking only at the excuses that apply to you. To do that would be to ignore my most important instruction, to read all of Chapters 1 to 8 in order. You will soon see that if you haven't used a particular excuse yet, you may have done so in the future. So without further ado, come with me as we totally shatter …

The **But** Syndrome

'But I can't because ... *I don't have the time*'

Of all of the excuses given as to why people don't eat well and exercise on a regular basis this is without question the one I hear the most – *"I would do, but I just don't have the time."* It's funny that the same people who say they don't have the time to look after themselves seem to be able to tell you exactly what's happening in *EastEnders, Coronation Street, Emmerdale* and *Big Brother*! They have the time to watch God knows how much TV, nip to the pub for a couple of hours a day, spend ages queuing for a 'hip and trendy' coffee, yet seemingly don't have the time to go for a walk or prepare an apple!

The one thing which we are all equal in is time. Every single one of us has access to 24 hours in a day and, no matter how busy we all *think* we are, we can always find time to eat well and exercise. It's simply down to priorities. It's like those people who say, "I didn't have time to call you", but what they really mean is "I didn't have time to call YOU". If someone had said, "here's a number and if you call it the person on the other end of the phone will give you 1 million pounds", I can guarantee they'd find the time.

Money Rich – Time Poor

You've got to ask yourself just how important you regard your health and well-being and where it fits into your priorities of life. Health and fitness should, without question, be at number one. It should be the very first thing you focus on above anything else, as without the correct nutrition and a good supply of oxygen you are not going to perform at your best. But more and more we are seeing a situation where people are Money Rich and Time Poor; or more accurately, Money Rich – Health Poor. The question really is, what's the point of earning all that money if it gives you a heart attack in the process? What's the point of trying to create a better tomorrow for your children if you don't have the energy to play with them *today*? There's nothing wrong with earning money, or working hard – I'm all for it – but it doesn't mean you can't look after your body at the same time.

I do realize that time for many people is becoming harder and harder to come by, but the point I'm making is that despite how much we rush around like headless chickens giving the impression to the world and ourselves that we are non-stop busy from morning till night, very rarely is that actually the case.

If we cut through the rubbish we tell ourselves, time is *not* the reason why we don't get the body and supreme health we crave. Time is simply yet another excuse people can give themselves to try to justify why they aren't healthy and don't have the body of their dreams. But again how much time does it actually take to rustle up a few stir-fried veggies, steam a bit of fish, make a delicious fresh juice or peel a banana? How much time does it really take to go for a walk, run or jump on a mini-trampoline? How much time do you need to push some weights? Yes, it may take some degree of effort to do the exercise part of things and, yes, you 'can't be bothered', but that's nothing to do with time. Please don't delude yourself any longer into thinking you can't do it because of time; we can all make the time if we want to enough.

If you have to be up for a flight at 4am to take you to paradise – you find the time. If someone close to you gets ill and you need to drop things to get to hospital – you find the time. If you crave chocolate and must have some NOW! – you find the time to go and get some. The point is if something's important enough to you – you find the time. The problem is, up until now, your health, body shape and well-being haven't been important enough to you. You may think they have, as like most people what you eat and how you look probably dominate a large part of your life – but you haven't wanted it enough. You haven't wanted it more than that tub of ice-cream for example!

Remember, if you want to turbo-charge your life, excuses have to go out of the window and not having enough time is just like all the other excuses we come up with as to why we can't exercise and eat well – complete bull-shit!

'But ... *I can't afford to get healthy*'

When it comes to your health, the truth is you cannot afford *not* to do it. I mean, how much is your heart worth? What about your kidneys or your liver, or how about your life? You cannot put a price on health. Four members of my family have died of cancer. All these people would gladly have given every penny they had for a body clear of cancer. It's times like these when people see clearly that money means nothing compared with health, and start wishing they had taken care of their bodies earlier.

My number one priority is to make certain I have good quality 'live' nutrients flowing through my system on a daily basis, no matter what the cost. Fortunately, despite what you may think, it doesn't cost any more to be healthy than it does to get sick. In reality, it's often cheaper! Regardless of your income, *everyone* can afford to exercise and get healthy.

How much does it actually cost to buy a bag of fruit or get up and go for a walk? It's funny how the same people who say they can't afford to eat well and exercise seem to find money for cigarettes, alcohol, going out and junk food. The average drinker will now spend in the region of £100,000 on alcohol in their lifetime; an average 20-a-day smoker will get through £65,000.

People think that getting fit and healthy means joining an expensive gym or buying organic ingredients, but you don't *need* those things to get fit and healthy.

All you need is a pair of trainers, plenty of water, some nutrient-rich foods and the right mental attitude.

Even juicing fruits and vegetables doesn't need to be expensive. Anyone can nip down to their local market at the end of the day when bargains are plentiful.

Despite what we have been conditioned to believe, we don't require a large quantity of food to thrive. One of the main reasons people overeat is because their bodies are suffering from malnutrition and 'false hungers'. When you burden your system with loads of junk food, your body will try its level best to extract whatever it can in order to survive. With so few nutrients contained within each plateful, the body soon cries out for more. This is why when you begin supplying your body with the 'live' nutrients it craves, you will find that you eat much less yet feel more satisfied.

'But there's nothing I can do about it because ...
fat is in my genes'

You may have fat in your jeans; but not in your genes! Of all the bullshit excuses I've heard as to why people can't lose weight, this has to go in at number one. It is true that depending on your genes you can have a *pre-disposition* for many illnesses including weight gain, but this doesn't mean you can't do anything about it.

My father didn't give me much, but one of the things he was generous with was his buggered-up genes. He managed to pass on a predisposition for asthma, eczema, psoriasis, hay fever and weight gain – nice! This means it takes less wrongdoing for me to get these ailments than some-one who is not predisposed to them. So yes, if your mother or father was overweight then it might be possible – unlikely, but possible – that they have passed on a gene which makes you gain weight easily. However, unlike asthma, eczema, psoriasis and hay fever, all of which can have other contributing factors, weight gain is *only* caused by one thing – eating too much of the wrong kinds of foods and not moving your body enough. People often say, 'My mother was fat so that's why I'm fat,' but chances are that's not even down to a predisposition; it's simply that they lived in the same house, ate the same food and watched the same amount of TV.

If you really want success on the slim, trim and energy-driven front, and have been hiding behind the rather convenient 'but it's in my genes' excuse, you'd better face up to the fact that once again it's all rubbish!

I don't care who you are. If I were to put you on what I call the David Blaine diet, where you are elevated in a glass box near Tower Bridge for 44 days with nothing to eat or drink except water, trust me, you'd lose weight. Equally, if I put you on a diet consisting only of water-rich live foods, fresh fish, lean white meat and freshly extracted 'live' juices, trust me again – you'd lose weight.

The predisposition for fat may indeed be in the genes of *some* people, but to suggest for a millisecond that even if these people ate well *and* exercised daily that their genes would prevent them from losing excess weight is absolute rubbish. I am so confident on this issue that I am willing to be challenged by anyone in the medical profession who thinks otherwise.

no more excuses!

This programme does work ... if *you* stop the bullshit excuses and just *do* it.

'But I don't understand it because ... *I never eat anything*'

I'm sure you've all heard this one. People who are the size of a house complaining about the fact they have got that way by complete fluke as they 'really don't eat that much'. You may be able to be a secret smoker, but it's very hard to eat in secret if you are predisposed to weight gain – IT SHOWS!

I'm teasing slightly as not everyone who is overweight is scoffing their way through bucketloads of chocolates and chips, but to say 'I don't eat anything or very little' is usually about a mile from the truth. It's true that many people don't realize how much they are eating. After all, if you eat anything standing up or from someone else's plate, it doesn't count! This is why when someone writes down what they eat over a week it often comes as a massive surprise. The problem is that many people often reach for food out of sheer habit, so the conscious brain doesn't take it in.

I think people genuinely believe that they 'don't eat that much', but this is only because they delude themselves. Often they're part of the, 'I don't usually but ...' gang. You know, the group of people who are always saying, 'I don't usually but ... *it's a special occasion*' or 'I don't usually but ... *oh why not*'. When you add them up, the 'I don't usuallys' soon mean a hell of a lot of extra calories. I'm not saying that after you read this book you won't genuinely have the 'I don't usually but what the hell it's a special occasion' moments (we are all human after all!). I'm just saying that if you are overweight and have somehow deluded yourself into thinking you really don't eat much, just write down EVERYTHING that passes your lips for a week and I think the evidence will be clear.

You've also got to remember that it's not just food which causes weight to stay on. Sugar-loaded drinks also play a massive part. If you are eating three balanced meals a day *and* drinking 2 litres of fizzy pop then you're not going to see a great deal of movement (on every level!).

Stop deluding yourself. If you are overweight you are clearly eating too much for *your* body's needs.

If you believe you can do nothing about your problem you will sit around getting fatter and sicker until the magic weight-loss pill has been found. The magic pill is in your mind, and once you stop the excuses and use the power of your mind, success is there for the taking.

'But it's much harder for me because ... *I've got a* *slow metabolism*,

Yes, you'd probably like to think so. This is one excuse I used to use all the time, and I honestly thought it was true ... *to some degree at least.*

One of the biggest myths about metabolic rate is that some people who are overweight have a slower metabolism than their slim friends.

They believe it's this 'fact', and not their intake of food and drink, which is causing their inability to lose those excess pounds. However, the reality is the complete opposite. The heavier you are, the *faster* your metabolic rate. Heavier people actually burn more calories than lighter people. This makes sense when you think about it, as it obviously takes more energy to move a heavier body than a lighter one.

It may seem that because of your metabolism, 'you only have to look at food' to gain weight. I'm afraid the truth is that if you only looked at it, all would be well!

I will repeat this until I'm blue in the face –

Eating too much of the wrong kinds of food and not moving your body enough on a regular basis are the only true reasons why people are overweight.

Not NASA stuff I know, but that's about it. It has not a jot to do with your metabolism – glad that's clear.

'But I've tried it all before and ... *it doesn't work for me*'

I was desperately trying to come up with another word to the one I'm going to use but there is simply no other word in the English language that captures what I want to say in response to this excuse – bollocks!

People who say, 'I've tried it all before' and 'nothing works for me' are basically talking rubbish. However, they've probably said it to so many people – and to themselves – so often that they have started to believe it.

What they really mean of course is, 'I've failed to follow what was being suggested', but of course you'll never hear that. All you'll hear is a load of excuses as to why that particular programme has failed *them*.

Just like the 'but it's in my genes' excuse, this one doesn't wash.

It doesn't matter who you are, or how big or small you are. If you eat nature's superfoods, move your body until you sweat on a regular basis, do some resistance training, think positively and get some fresh air – 'IT' will work.

The truth is there is no 'IT' – IT IS YOU! 'It' will work if you do 'it'. If you fail to do it, then IT hasn't failed – YOU HAVE! If you want success, if you really want to take charge of your health and your life, you must understand that you'll never have the body or life of your dreams if you keep coming up with 'but', 'but', 'but'.

'But it's hard for me because ... I eat as a response to emotion'

So many people believe that they will never be able to change because they are 'emotional eaters', and as life will always be full of emotion, what's the point of even trying to change? On the surface this may seem true – again, I would often use this as an excuse – but once looked at, it just doesn't wash.

You may well think that you are one of those people who eat purely as a response to emotion, but I will tell you now that you eat *certain things* as a response to emotion. I've never heard anyone saying, 'I'm really pissed off today. I need a grape'! People never turn to things like steamed fish and stir-fired veggies when they're bored or upset. When people look to feed an emotion they always turn to 'foods' containing refined sugars, fats or a combination of the two, such as chocolate, fast food, muffins, bagels, cakes, breads and ice cream.

People 'use' refined fats and sugars in much the same way as people 'use' drugs, and the excuses for taking them are pretty much the same.

If you ask a smoker why they are smoking they may say it's because they're bored, stressed, relaxed, sad, happy, lonely, anxious, angry, excited, upset, nervous, and so on. In fact, there doesn't seem to be an emotion which isn't in some way linked to their smoking. If you ask a cocaine addict to come up with 'reasons' as to why they are taking that drug, you will hear the same list of emotional excuses and the same goes for heroin, crack and other drugs. The fact that most of the emotional excuses completely contradict one another doesn't seem to occur to those trying to justify their actions. Equally, those getting their fixes from refined sugars and fats will also blame any number of emotions:

- ■ 'I ate the chocolate bar because I didn't get the job and was consoling myself'
- ■ 'I ate the chocolate bar because I did get the job and was celebrating'

People eat rubbish food when they're sad *and* when they're happy, when they are stressed *and* when they are relaxed; when they're bored *and* when they're 'on the run'. The sad truth is they have been saying how certain foods help certain emotions for so long that, like smokers and other drug takers, they have ended up believing what they're saying; but it's all nonsense. If you're bored you can shove as many cakes in your face as you like but you'll still be bored. If you're upset, all the ice cream in the world will never console you. If you're stressed, squashing a large piece of pizza in your mouth will not calm you down and if you're feeling lonely, eating bucketloads of rubbish foods will not fill the gap in your life. In fact, not only will your emotions not be helped *at all* by eating drug-like refined sugars and fats, but on top of the boredom, stress, loneliness or whatever, you will now have to deal with feeling guilty, anxious and fat!

What would you think if you saw a monkey stuffing loads of rubbish food into its mouth and then trying to explain its actions by saying, 'I'm a bit anxious today'? Yes, you'd think, 'stone me, a talking monkey'! But seriously, wild animals have more stress and more anxiety on a daily basis than we are ever likely to experience. Now you may well argue with that, but often their lives are a 24/7 battle to find something to eat or to stop themselves being eaten. You may have to pay your bills, go to a job you don't like, or have to put up with traffic for hours on end – but you probably know exactly where your next meal is coming from and you're not about to be eaten! Imagine how much *more* stressful and anxious wild animals' lives would be if they had substances entering their system which created *additional* feelings of stress and anxiety to the ones they are already experiencing.

People who consume rubbish foods and drinks all the time are more stressed and anxious than people who don't.

This is because refined fats, sugars and drinks like caffeine all create empty withdrawal-type symptoms which are similar to normal emotions like anxiety, stress and boredom. Like drug addicts, people then try to deaden those feelings with more of the same. *Initially*, the refined junkie foods appear to help, but that's only because they have taken the edge off a low caused by the last dose.

You cannot feed an emotional hunger with food – you can only feed a physical hunger. Anything you eat when not genuinely physically hungry will be stored as fat!

I will explain more about this in the Seven Deadly Dietary Sins (page 106), but for now, if you keep saying you are an 'emotional eater', please stop the bullshit and remove this 'but' from your life.

'But, do you know what? ... I'm "fine" as I am'

Fine, which of course stands for:

Freaked-out Insecure Neurotic & Emotional

Most of the time when you ask people 'How are you?' and get the response 'I'M FINE, thank you', it usually means they're feeling either 'Freaked-out', 'Insecure', 'Neurotic', 'Emotional' or a combination of the lot. 'How's your diet going?' 'Oh, fine' – meaning 'It's making me feel insecure, I'm getting a touch neurotic about the whole thing, I'm a bit emotional and it's beginning to freak me out – so as you can see, I'm fine!'

I don't know about you, but I don't want to spend my life feeling 'fine'. I don't even want to just feel 'good', although good is clearly better than fine. I want to feel pretty damn incredible most of the time, or as my good friend Martin says, 'outstanding'.

The problem is most people settle for a life of 'fine' or 'alright'. 'How's your relationship with your partner?' – 'Oh, fine.' 'How are your finances?' – 'Oh, fine.' 'How's your health?' – 'Oh, fine.' 'How's your job?' – 'Oh, fine'. 'How's your life?' – 'Oh you know, it's OK, it's alright … I'm FINE!'

The idea behind turbo-charging your life in 14 days is to move way beyond settling for a level of health and vitality and a body that's simply 'alright' or 'fine' – it's about setting ourselves new standards, raising our expectations of ourselves on a daily basis.

'But it's hard because ... *I have children*'

It doesn't matter if you have one child or a football team's worth; there is no reason on the planet why having children should prevent you from eating well and exercising.

Why does having kids, even being a single parent, prevent you from eating some fruit, making a juice or doing some exercise? And why does having kids mean you have to stuff your face?

When you think about it, it surely takes longer to make toast and cereal than it does to prepare a delicious melon – there's even less washing up!

But the minute you say something like that you get hit with another but; 'But it's difficult because you have to make food for the kids.' Yes, and so what? It is true that you do have to make the kids' food, but you don't *have* to make them unhealthy food, and even if you have little terrorists who rule the roost in terms of what's for dinner, why does this prevent you from making a healthy meal for yourself? In fact, having children gives you a reason to shop and prepare for mealtimes.

If you say you are unhealthy, overweight and lethargic because you have children, you are inadvertently blaming their being born for your health demise.

Yet, if you think back, your eating, drinking and exercise habits might not have been exactly fantastic before you gave birth. Whatever, you still need to understand that it's not the children preventing you from getting the body you crave – it's only you and your excuses!

'But I can't make it to the gym as I'm at home with the kids all day.' Again, so what? This doesn't stop you exercising or eating well. You can get some kind of home exercise equipment, take the kids to the park, go for a walk, etc.

There is always a way if you are committed, no matter how many children you are *fortunate* to have. If you really wanted to join a gym and make it there a few times a week – you could. If you really wanted to start eating well – you could. Children are a blessing; it's time to stop blaming them for your bad habits.

'But the kids like McDonald's so it's hard'

I was on the phone to a friend of a friend recently about a matter which had nothing to do with health. Because of what I do, however, health, and in particular his weight, soon came into the conversation. He said, 'If you are what you eat, then I'm a Big Mac,' and proceeded to tell me how his eating habits had gone pear-shaped (or burger-shaped) because of his son. I asked him how on earth he worked that out. His reply was one I'd heard a few times, 'Well, he loves McDonald's and I have to take him in there.''And?' I replied. 'And, you know, once you're in there …'

Firstly, what does he mean, he *has* to take him there? Does his son have a gun to his head? Is his son in charge? Isn't this man meant to be his child's guardian? Isn't he meant to be looking out for his child's best interest even if that means having to be a strong parent and say no? After all, if your child wanted to go and play in quicksand because it looked fun, you'd shout, scream and do whatever it took to make sure they never went in: you certainly wouldn't join them because they're doing it. Why do so many people these days have such difficulty in saying a simple NO to their children? Some people see places like McDonald's as a treat, but that's hardly an argument.

If parents think a treat is to feed their loved ones a load of refined sugar and fat, then I'd hate to see what they do to punish them.

Secondly, even if he does see it as a treat and his son only has McDonald's once a week, why on earth does that mean he has to join his son with a Big Mac and fries? I explained that McDonald's now do salads, so he could always tuck into one of those. But of course the reason why he doesn't is the same reason why he doesn't say NO to his boy – *he* wants to go and *he* wants a McDonald's; but boy, aren't kids a great scapegoat for our failures?

Stop blaming the fact you've had kids or you've got kids; if you want a slim trim body you can get one. You don't have to feed your kids junk; you don't have to pander to their every terrorist tantrum for their next sugar fix and you can be strong and take control of at least their household's dietary habits. I realize that some households are different and many 'buts' can come into play. 'But I'm only the step-parent so I must feed them what their real parent wants', 'but my kids are teenagers and they are so set in their ways it would be wrong to change now', or whatever. If that's the case then it still doesn't mean you have to eat stuff from their plates and it doesn't mean because they eat junk food that it automatically means you have to.

You might see a great opportunity to add another but, something like 'but I can't make it to the gym as I'm at home with the kids all day'. Again so what? This doesn't stop you exercising or eating well. You can get some kind of home exercise equipment; take the kids to the park; go for a walk; etc. etc. Remember the question should always be 'What could I do in this situation to move more towards my goal?' It's a great question; it stops the 'buts' and your brain will always think of a solution. Ask the right questions and you get the right answers

There is always a way if you are committed. There is always a way if you really make it a priority – no matter how many children you are *fortunate* to have. If you really wanted to join a gym and make it there a few times a week – you could. If you really wanted to start eating well – you could; if you wanted to get the children involved in playing every night or joining some kind of active sports club – you could. Children are a blessing; it's time to stop blaming them for your bad habits.

'But it's different for me because ... *I know it all already*'

This is one 'but' I love. When it comes to the subject of health and fitness, because there have been so many 'diet' books, God knows how many TV shows about this subject and because food plays such a role in today's Western world, everyone is an expert. The amount of people I see who at first say, 'I know that' or 'tell me something I don't know' is amazing. What's amazing is in many cases they do know it all (well, most of it anyway). They know that if they eat less junk, increase their intake of fruit and veg and take regular exercise they will change body shape, have more energy and be healthier. More and more people are also aware of the danger of refined sugar and fat; how too much alcohol can cause weight gain and speed up the aging process; how sitting around on furniture for hours on end can cause bone and back problems; and people are even becoming experts on how certain foods have a low or high 'GI' (Glycaemic Index) rating and what role that plays on fat levels in their body. In fact with more and more 'health' and 'diet' books hitting the shops and becoming number-one bestsellers throughout the western world, I think it's safe to say more and more people aren't just getting to know a little bit more about how certain foods act on the body – they really are becoming experts in this field.

I think it is almost undisputed that most people, even if they don't know the exact science behind certain foods and drinks, have a pretty good idea of what's best to eat for a healthy lifestyle. But just knowing it doesn't mean anything. I know that if I actually listen to the Spanish course I paid good money for that sits with dust on my top shelf, I'll be able to learn Spanish. But just knowing that doesn't mean I'll ever do it. Just knowing what to eat and what exercises you need to do to get the body of your dreams means jack unless you are going to actually get off your derrière and do it.

Even the Experts have Buts!

Another problem for people is that many of the true diet experts aren't exactly applying what they teach and often aren't exactly the picture of health themselves. Many seem to have the old doctor adage of 'do as I say not as I do'. It is amazing how many people seem happy to take health advice from unhealthy people. It is true that you don't necessarily need to be the best football player in order to be a good football manager, but at the same time I personally would never take financial advice from a poor person and I wouldn't go to a stop-smoking therapist who had a cigarette hanging out of their mouth. I think I make my point!

What I'm saying is, knowing what's good and bad and being an 'expert' on the subject of health and fitness doesn't mean anything unless you apply it to your own life. After all what's the point of being the most knowledgeable health and fitness expert if you're fat and ill yourself?

I'm not so much here to teach you what to eat, drink and how to exercise for optimum health and vitality – although clearly these nuggets are covered in depth in case of any doubt and you'll have a step-by-step plan for the 14-day Turbo Charge Your Life programme – but it's more to show you how to *apply* the knowledge which most of you already have. It's designed to show exactly what is needed to get off of your butt and catapult your life to a new level. Remember, *knowing* what to do is one thing, but *doing* what you know is what makes the big difference between those who talk a good game and those who are actually in the game.

'But I don't really need to change as ... I'm only a little overweight'

Not everyone reading this book is overweight. Some are underweight and some are slim but have no energy and bad eating and drinking habits. However, for those who are overweight – and I mean overweight – but have for years been saying things like 'I'm a little overweight' or 'I could do with losing a few pounds here and there', please let me say what all those you come into contact with are thinking and saying behind your back – you are not a little overweight:

YOU ARE **FAT!**

Not only are you fat, but as is the way of the world, your character is also called into question, and you can add the words 'git' and 'bastard' after fat to get a true picture of what's being said.

I realize that sounds harsh, but until you see things as they really are you will never make the change.

If you continue to make the situation seem better than it is then what possible motivation would you have for change?

I realize that in some cases people saying to you out loud 'you fat bastard' isn't exactly useful, and could have you locking yourself in a room with half a hundred weight of cake and ice cream in order to 'comfort' yourself. However, if you are constantly being real about the situation, and if you no longer hide behind things like 'I'm just a tad tubby' or avoid looking in the mirror, then your brain will feel more and more frustrated about the current situation and try to do something about it.

When I was at school I was nicknamed 'Fatty Vale', and every day I would get picked on for being overweight. My mother and all the people who cared about me said things like, 'It's just a bit of puppy fat', and 'You're not fat, just a little tubby', but with children you get the truth. They tell it as it really is and, yes, I was indeed 'Fatty Vale'. This constant barrage of verbal abuse led me to go from Fatty Vale who couldn't run a bath and was always last at cross-country to a person who just 12 weeks later was Slim Vale who not only finished the cross-country course on time, but even broke the school record for that distance!

I was not willing to be called Fatty Vale again and from that point on (when I was 13) until I left school at 15 I was never fat again, and I never got detention for being late after cross-country. As soon as I left school, however, I discovered beer, bar snacks, the kebab shop and video games, and was Fatty Vale again before you knew it. Only this time I didn't have people coming up to me everyday telling me so; they just did it behind my back.

So please, if you are very overweight – and I mean 20 pounds or more over what you should be – get real with your situation and understand fully what people are saying. You are not overweight, you are not a little 'rotund' and you are not 'big boned'. Use the 'F' word – you are FAT! And as such you are at *huge* risk of developing heart disease, diabetes or one of the other major debilitating illnesses as well as having to live your daily life in a body with little energy that brings you down.

'But I'm fed up with having to conform ... *big is beautiful and I'm fat and happy*'

This is another excuse I hear over and over again. When all else fails, tell the world the reason why you don't change is because you don't actually want to. In reality, *all* women would love to be slim, and *all* men would love some definition and at least a four pack – that's just how it is.

Women love to buy weekly magazines with picture after picture of celebrities with something wrong with them. If Britney gets a spot, or Cameron Diaz has some cellulite, then all of a sudden the world seems a brighter place. I know it's hard for women to believe, but nowadays men do exactly the same. If David Beckham were to ever get a few spots or, heaven forbid, get fat, most of the men in the country would be jumping for joy. This is because it's much easier to drag someone else down in order to try to make yourself look better than it is to put in the effort to lift your own world. Many people don't even do this consciously and there's no malice involved; it's just they've done it for so long and, given we also have a culture that does it readily, it appears normal.

Fat is Not Attractive

People can say that many years ago, being fat was seen as a sign of wealth and regarded as sexy, and they can even harp on about how in many cultures it still is today, but that doesn't change how it is in the West here and now. If we're being frank, and I believe we are, someone who is fat is not as pleasing to the eye as someone who is slim.

In today's politically correct world, that statement will have some people ranting and raving and reaching for the nearest cream bun, but if we cut through the crap – it's true. If it wasn't, then people like Dawn French would be used to advertise the latest Ferrari rather than chocolate! I don't think anyone could look at Dawn French and say she isn't a beautiful-looking woman. My point is that if she's beautiful as she is, she would be *stunning* if she were slim.

'But that's shallow – beauty comes from within.' Yes I agree, and in an ideal world people would be able to see the inner beauty in everyone. However, having been fat and suffered from severe psoriasis in the past, I know first hand that most of the world isn't like that.

They say personality goes a long way, but in some cases it can never stretch that far!

And talking of personality, it's not just coincidence that you often see 'fat and jolly' people. We have to make the best of what we've got, and if your external shell isn't what the world likes to see, you tend to develop more of a personality. This is why some models seem to have had major personality bypasses. They haven't had to develop that side of themselves to attract people; often they just need to walk into a room and people come running.

I know it's not fair and I know it shouldn't be this way – *but it is!* I didn't make the rules and neither did you, but if you're in this 'game of life' and you want to get the best out of it, we have to accept some of them. There is of course one huge advantage when you have been overweight and then lose it: you end up with a slim, trim body *and* a personality!

If people genuinely thought being overweight was a good thing then they would actively encourage their children to overeat and get fat, but if you ask any parent if they want their child to be slim or fat, they opt for slim every time.

This is not just for health reasons but also so that they're not picked on by their peers and have the energy to really enjoy their life.

Those people who say, 'I'm fat and happy' may well be just that, fat and happy – but this doesn't mean they're happy *because* they're fat. It also doesn't mean they wouldn't be a damn site happier if they were slim. If you feel there's nothing you can do about a particular situation, like being fat in this case, you have no real alternative but to try and justify why you are the way you are. Because no one wants to look as though they are weak-willed jelly fish who cannot control their eating, it seems easier to say, 'I'm happy the way I am, I don't want to change.' But the reality is that's a load of old tosh as *everyone* who's fat, regardless of what they say out loud, would love to wake up in a slim, trim, energy-driven body. It's only when they have exhausted all other possible 'excuses' that they come out with the 'I don't want to change' line; after all how can anyone possibly argue with that? If they don't want to change and are happy as they are – good for them! But in truth they are not as happy as Larry as they are, despite what they say; they would love to change. The saddest part about the 'I'm fat and happy line' is that the person saying it has almost resigned themselves to a life of 'fat'. They have no doubt already 'tried' God knows how many diets and are now convinced they're beyond hope. This leads to a need to justify why they are not doing anything about their weight and health, 'I'm fat and I'm happy' usually being the outcome. If you are fat and genuinely think it's beautiful and are genuinely happy, then I for one am happy for you – I don't believe you, but I'm happy for you. The fact is, though, if all was well in fat land you wouldn't be reading this book. I know what it's like to be fat and I know what it's like to be slim – and guess what? Give me slim any day!

'But It's All Down to the Magazines'

Some people even have the gall to blame the glossy magazines for being overweight and unhealthy. They claim if it wasn't the pressure to conform they wouldn't rebel and eat. What amazes me is the people who bitch about these magazines buy them all the time. I know this may sound stupidly easy but if you think the magazines are causing your problem – *don't buy them!* But they do prove my theory that fat is not the new black. If it were, we wouldn't have pictures of nice-looking bodies on the front covers of magazines, we would have fat people. People like to look at attractive people – that's just how it is.

But the main reason why 'big isn't beautiful' is because when you're big you just don't *feel* beautiful – you feel fat and bloated, you can't move as you want; you can't wear what you want and you don't feel as sexy as you want. There is nothing beautiful about a life spent feeling that way and with disease hanging over your head.

'**But** I have an injury so ... *I can't exercise*'

You must have heard them (you may even be one them) – people who say the reason they got overweight and unfit was because they sprained their foot, knackered their elbow, broke their leg or damaged their ligaments, and so the list goes on and on. However, in order to have an injury so severe that it stops you from doing any kind of exercise you would need to be in a Christopher Reeve situation. Actually, that's not even true. One of the many things the truly remarkable Christopher Reeve did for the nine years of his life as a paraplegic was to make sure he exercised when-ever he could. His exact words from his inspirational book *Nothing Is Impossible* are, 'I've also found the self-discipline to exercise when I don't feel like it ...' Remember these words if you've ever banged on about how you can't exercise because of whatever.

If you have a leg injury, do some upper-body exercises. If you can't move your arms, move your legs. If you can't put pressure on your joints, go for a swim or jump on a trampoline. If you really can't move *anything* without being in pain, do some deep-breathing exercises and cut down on your fuel consumption. After all, you wouldn't put the same amount of fuel into your car if you weren't using it as much as usual, would you?

There isn't any reason on the planet why anyone should become unhealthy or overweight just because they have an injury. I've seen people in wheelchairs whacking tennis balls over nets and shooting basketballs into hoops, and I've seen people with no arms running marathons. In fact, I've seen people with no legs running marathons with prosthetic limbs.

Whatever the injury, it shouldn't be an excuse for not achieving your health and body-shape goals. Look at someone like Tanni Gray Thompson, a truly remarkable and superb athlete. Losing the use of her legs didn't stop her training and getting the rest of her body super-fit, so much so that she has, at the time of writing, won an incredible 11 gold medals for Great Britain at the Paralympics. What's your excuse?

Then you have the, 'But I used to ...' gang. You know, the people who tell you how much sport they *used* to play; how they *used* to run all the time and how they *used* to always be in the gym. But so what? Used to means Jack! You can spend your life living in the 'what I used to be able to do' world, but that's not going to change how you look and feel today.

The truth is most people can usually exercise with an injury, no matter what the situation. There is always a way if the person is committed. Instead of looking at what isn't possible because of the injury, people should focus on what *can* be done.

'But you've got to live ... *you could get run over by a bus next week*'

That's true – but don't you want the week to be nice before the bus comes along?

For every action there is always a reaction and every action you take today has a knock-on effect which will determine your tomorrow. People who are overweight didn't get that way *one day*; it took many months and years of consuming too much of the wrong kinds of foods and drinks and not moving their bodies very much to get that way. It's all very well and good living as if there's no tomorrow and saying, 'the bomb could go off tomorrow' or 'I could get run over by a bus tomorrow', but what happens when it doesn't and you don't? What happens when you eat and drink junk every day, get fat, unhealthy and lethargic – or all three – only to wake up and find that tomorrow very much did happen and it's here to face today? I used to make the excuse that 'Anything could happen tomorrow, so why not just indulge', only to find that 'tomorrow' *always* happened and I would still have to face it as a fat, unhealthy bastard!

Yes, you may get run over by a bus next week, but what about today? Don't you want to feel good *today*? Don't you want to be able to wear what you want *today*? Don't you want to wake up with energy and vibrancy *today*? Don't you want to feel light and slim *today*? Those people who say they are eating and drinking junk *because* they are 'living for today' or because the bomb could go off tomorrow seem to have missed the irony. It's all about today, and the only way to create a much better today is by understanding that there *is* a tomorrow. Unless you keep an eye on tomorrow it's going to come up and bite you on the bum, and that could be one hell of a bum!

This excuse, like all of the others, is total rubbish.

Nobody, when they are tucking into a cream bun and a large Coke, is ever thinking, 'The only reason I'm doing this is in case something happens to me tomorrow.' If you really thought tomorrow wasn't coming, the last thing on your mind would be, 'Yippee, how much junk food can I stuff down my gullet today?' Your only focus would be on finding the people you love and telling them how you feel.

'But Jason, life is too short.' I agree, life is too short, and unless you change it will be even shorter! It's also too short not to live your dreams; it's too short to live feeling sluggish and overweight, hating the way you look and feel; it's too short to be scared to get into a bathing costume; it's too short to hit your head on the pillow every night *hoping* things will be different tomorrow; it's too short to wake up every day with a junk-food hangover; it's too short to collapse at the end of the working day with only enough energy to slump in front of the TV for hours on end – YES, LIFE IS TOO SHORT – so stop saying, 'I could get run over by a bus tomorrow' because that's *not* why you eat and drink rubbish or don't exercise – it's just another excuse.

I suppose there is some argument on the other side though. I mean, if you keep eating and drinking rubbish and end up as big as a house, the chances of a bus actually being able to run you over would be pretty slim!

'But I can't because ... *I'm too old*'

Too old for what exactly? Too old to buy some fruit and veg? Too old to peel a banana? Too old to go for a walk? Too old to push some vegetables through a juicer and drink it? Or too old to live?

The truth is that if you believe you're too old then you're right, and if you believe you're not too old you're also right.

I'm not saying that the years don't take their toll. As we get older we often genuinely can't do what we used to be capable of, but it doesn't mean for a second we are washed up and on the scrapheap. Age is just another excuse, which once again is simply based on fear – the fear of taking the leap from settling for what we have to making life an unbelievable adventure.

Two ladies in their sixties attended one of our Ultimate Health Weekends. Having read my first book, *Slim 4 Life*, a few months earlier, they had decided to get up and, as one of the chapters suggests, Get Busy Living. In the time since they had read the book, and, more importantly, acted upon it, they experienced not only an increase in physical energy but found their worlds expanded by the day. On this particular weekend they played 'net-football' on the beach at 7am; swam in a cold, but beautiful lake first thing on a Sunday morning; climbed an enormous height up a pole onto a platform where they then attached themselves to a Zip-Slide and slid James Bond-style down a mountain; completed a 50ft high-ropes assault course; ate and drank pure live foods; and joined in with everything. I know people in their thirties who wouldn't have the physical or mental energy to do that.

It's not about your chronological age, it's about your *mental* age, i.e. how youthful you are in the mind and how much zest and spirit you have for life.

I met a young man on holiday and asked if he wanted to come 'wake-boarding' with me (this is like snowboarding but on water with a boat pulling you along). He seemed unsure, so I told him that if he had done any snowboarding or skateboarding it would be an advantage. His eyes lit up and he explained that skateboarding was his passion. When I asked if he still did it, he said, 'Oh not now, I gave it up as I'm getting too old to do that sort of thing.' I asked him how old he was, and he was 29! He thought it looked silly for a 29-year-old to be on a skate-board. Who gives a flying 360-degree jump?

You cannot possibly let *your* thoughts of what other people *may* think of you dictate how you live your life.

If I want to skateboard at 99 let alone 29 then I will! Stopping physical passions cause people to 'age' before their time.

When ex-veteran Ray Sheriff jumped from an aeroplane with the Red Devils on 18 September 2004 he was 84, and he was blind! He was just one of ten men aged between 79 and 85 that made the jump in order to commemorate the battle of Arnhem. He has made the jump in the same place, on the same date, every year since he was 70. Ray lost his sight in a German mortar attack in World War II, but being blind and 84 years of age isn't enough to produce one 'but' from this amazing man.

Life begins at 40 ... or 50, 60, 70, 80 or whenever you want it to.

Life begins when you say, 'That's it. I'm no longer going to sit and be a spectator of life – I'm going to get off of my backside and live a little.' It's when you aren't willing to settle for a mindset which falsely tells you 'you're too old' or 'you've had your time so it's time to sit back now'. We are on this planet for a short enough time as it is; the last thing you want is to tell yourself you're too old for anything.

Some people don't think they're too old; they think that they're either too overweight or have battered their inner organs so much that it's just not worth making the change as it's too late. But the human body is one of the most rejuvenating survival machines on the planet and no matter how much we've battered it over the years, the second we give it the opportunity to heal, it will do everything within its power to make optimum health possible. No matter how 'old' you are, or what condition or conditions you have; if you supply the body with the right tools – 'live' foods, drinks and physical movement – it will do whatever it can to breed life and vitality to your body and mind.

'But I've tried juicing and ... *it's such a hassle!*'

Before I get on to why this excuse doesn't wash, I want to stress that **THIS IS NOT A JUICING BOOK!** Yes, juicing will play a part during the 14-day programme. The chances are, once you start to live, feel and see the difference juicing makes, you will continue well beyond that time. However, the main focus of this book is to show you how to drop the bullshit excuses.

The same people who say it takes too long to make a juice and clean the machine don't seem to have the same misgivings when spending God knows how much time cooking bacon and eggs and cleaning the pan!

Once again, it's all about priorities, and anyone can easily find the time to juice if they want.

It's hardly the most difficult process. All you need to do is pop a few fruits and veggies into the juicer and push down. How flipping tricky is that? Even cleaning the machine is hardly back-breaking work, is it? I mean, all you have to do is rinse a couple of parts and spend about one minute (if that) cleaning the filter part – so big deal. Most juicers will now even go into the dishwasher, making juicing life even easier.

Millions of people all over the world would kill for the opportunity to have the liquid fuel contained within fresh fruits and vegetables feeding every cell in their body. These are people who often walk 20 miles a day to find water. Somehow I don't think they'd moan a great deal if they 'had' to juice the finest fruits and vegetables from around the world.

Juicing can be super fast – if you know what you are doing.

In reality, it shouldn't take any longer than 10 minutes to make a juice *and* clean the machine. Like anything new, juicing takes a short while to get the hang of, so don't throw in the towel after just one attempt. No matter what, you will be juicing for at least 14 days during the programme, so even if you 'hate juicing' you can easily do it for 14 days.

'But it's hard for me because ... I'm *on the road all the time!*'

It is true that travelling makes it tricky, but don't think for a millisecond that you can't eat healthily or even do this programme when 'on the road'. Again, if someone said they'd give you a million pounds if you could find a way to eat healthily while 'on the road' – you'd soon find a way. It's not that you can't eat healthily when on the road; it's that you won't. It hardly takes a great deal of preparation to eat an apple on the go or to throw together a decent wholemeal sandwich for the journey; and there isn't a hotel or restaurant where you can't find something healthy to eat. After all, you can get fish, veg and salad almost anywhere.

I was once in the company of a man who had just written a book on weight loss and how easy it can be. Someone asked him, as politely as possible, why, if it was all so easy, he was himself, well, fat. He went on to try to explain that it was harder for him because he lived in Spain! Now why on earth living in Spain prevents you from eating well is a mystery to one and all, but this just proves that if someone wants to try to justify their eating they will say anything, no matter how ludicrous it may sound.

If you are 'on the road', instead of instantly saying, 'But I can't because ...' ask yourself an empowering 'but' – 'But what *could* I do to eat healthily while I'm away?' You will find that by asking that question, you will instantly give yourself a good chance of finding an answer. Remember, there is always a way if you stop the BS excuses and ask the right questions.

'But I can't even start because ... I don't have the energy'

On the surface this may appear true for many people. You may have bought this book because you want more energy. However, a lack of energy is no excuse for not getting nutritionally and physically fit. After all, how much energy does it take to pick up a piece of fruit and eat it? How much energy do you need to put some fish and veggies in a steamer and turn the knob? Even going for a long walk hardly requires the raw energy of Linford Christie, now does it?

You may not have *enough* energy to do various things you want, but eating well is not one of them. Once again, it's funny how the same people who don't have enough energy to prepare good food seem to find enough energy to get off the sofa and hit McDonald's or find their way to the pub!

The irony is that the *lack* of physical movement is a major cause of lethargy.

I will cover this point in greater depth later, but people who go to the gym will know that if they feel tired and hungry at the end of the day but somehow muster the energy to get to the gym, when they leave they're *less* hungry and *less* tired than before they went in. Why? Because by moving their body they have given a good blast of oxygen to their cells and have cleaned out a lot of the dead cells that have built up during the day. This leaves the person's system feeling lighter and their mind clearer, and gives them an overall feeling of *increased* energy. On top of that, because they've given their body a good dose of two of the primary human needs – oxygen and water – they are now *less* hungry.

Slim Chance

I was filming a documentary-style programme for Channel 5 entitled 'Fat Families – Slim Chance'. One of the mothers was a massive 27 stone (378 lb/171.5 kg) in weight and she was just 27 years old. Even worse, her daughter was 14½ stone (203 lb/92 kg) and she was just 9 years old! As you can imagine the mother – Michelle – had a suitcase full of excuses, but one excuse she couldn't make was she didn't have enough time. Time was one thing her entire family had plenty of. She didn't work and rarely left the house. In fact she hadn't even been to the supermarket herself for over 4 years! The first time I saw her I said, 'Right, we're going shopping to get some healthy stuff in.' Immediately it was met with a 'but I can't, because …' response. She claimed she couldn't go because she was tired *and* had a bad back. This is what I call a 'double but'. The more 'buts' a person has the bigger the health and fitness problem, and, of course, the bigger the actual butt!

Now if I thought she had had a back so bad that she really couldn't move then I would have left it. However, I've been in this business long enough to know that anyone that size didn't get that way without a million 'I can't, because …' excuses. The fact is that if at the end of the shopping trip someone had been there to reward her with a cheque for £100,000, she would have been skating round the aisles.

It's sad that most people will get excited about money but very rarely about their health, yet without health, without the confidence that a vibrant and trim body gives you, as I've already pointed out – you're poor.

'But What About M.E.?'

I realize that some people do have a genuine reason to feel lethargic; in particular I'm talking about M.E. and CFS (Chronic Fatigue Syndrome). Not everyone who has been diagnosed with M.E. or CFS genuinely has those conditions; many just have a lack of physical fitness and mental drive. However, for those who genuinely have these conditions they are certainly very real and drinking a few freshly extracted juices isn't going to cut the mustard. But again even those genuinely with M.E. and CFS don't have to let their illness control *every* aspect of their lives and having M.E. or CFS doesn't mean you can't do anything to help the situation. The biggest problem with those with M.E. and CFS is that they tend to say, 'But I can't as I have M.E.' before they say anything else. This often leads to a state of helplessness and a brain which in the end refuses to seek possible ways to improve the situation.

There is NO QUESTION that no matter what **the disease, if the person DOESN'T SMOKE**, drinks very **moderately, EATS WELL,** has a positive outlook and does their best **to do as much exercise as they can,** as well as **seeking out as much good air and sunshine as possible –** THEY WILL FEEL BETTER than if **they *didn't*** make any changes.

The truth is even if you have been diagnosed with either condition and you want to improve you must, like everyone else, stop the 'buts' and do everything within your power to help your situation.

'But what's the point ... I'll *never* look like Jennifer Aniston'

Yes, and I'll never look like Brad Pitt, but so what? It's not about looking like someone else, or being like someone else. It's about getting a better body shape for *you* and being a more vibrant *you*.

When I was fat and covered from head to toe with psoriasis, I used to look at people with good physiques and clear skin and dream of being them. What I was wishing for was not to be them, but a slim and clear-skinned me. I'm not exactly the best-looking biscuit in the barrel, and I certainly don't have a true six pack or a perfect body, but I'm a slimmer, trimmer version of my former self. I have the energy I need and I'm as happy as pie with it.

You may never look like Jennifer Aniston or Brad Pitt, but then neither will Jennifer or Brad. It's no secret that magazine pictures of glamorous celebrities are not exactly the real deal. Some of the best make-up artists, photographers, lighting experts and airbrush wizards have all played their part in making them look incredible. Don't get me wrong, Jennifer and Brad look good with a capital G and of course genes clearly played a part in this, but we should never want to be other people – we are all unique and we should always embrace that.

Never lose *you*. You are unique and you should ALWAYS want that *distinction*.

'But I don't need to change because ...
compared with most I'm *doing OK*'

One of the biggest mistakes people make is to compare themselves with other people in order to gauge their own success. But are they comparing themselves to people who are at their peak mental and physical condition, or to the masses who are suffering from overweight, lethargy and ill health, and who may end up with heart disease, cancer and an unfulfilled life?

Feel Like an *Instant Success* –
Hang Around with Losers!

The easiest way to feel like a good tennis player is to hang around with people who can't play as well as you; the easiest way to feel slim is to hang around with people fatter than you; and the easiest way to feel extremely healthy and full of energy is to hang around with people who are ill and can't move!

One of the easiest ways to feel 'OK' or to feel successful is by comparing yourself with those people who aren't doing as 'OK' as you. But just because you are doing 'OK' *compared to them*, it doesn't mean for a millisecond that you are actually doing OK.

That's a Bit OFF!

It's like the slim ... ish person who hangs around with people who are larger than they are – it's what I call the 'OFF' (Obligatory Fat Friend). Sure, compared to their fat friends they *seem* to be doing 'OK' on the weight and health front, but just because they are slimmer than their friends it doesn't mean they are not fat! It simply means that *compared to them* they are doing 'OK' and *compared to them* they are slim. But if you saw them on their own or up against some people at the peak of their physical fitness they would look fat and instantly feel that they weren't doing that 'OK' after all.

In the area of health it's so easy to feel good compared to most people. Heaven knows all you have to do is hit the gym a couple of times a week and eat a few pieces of fruit and you're already doing more 'OK' than most. But this may be nowhere near what *you* need for you to get the body of *your* dreams and energy levels *you* crave.

The only person you should ever compare yourself to is you. Only compare yourself to how good *you* can be in a particular area of *your* life, not how great you are compared with other people. You know what you are capable of and you know exactly what is needed for you to feel successful. Success cannot be gauged by money or even body shape; success is doing whatever it takes on a daily basis to truly live as opposed to exist. You can be slim and feel like a failure or overweight and feel like a success. Being a success is not the end result: success is a daily feeling; it's based on whether you feel you have done what it takes *today* to get your best *tomorrow* at the same time as enjoying the *present*. It's about hitting your head on the pillow at the end of the day feeling proud and fulfilled – that's true success.

We all have a choice and we can spend our lives doing just 'OK' or we can decide to step up a level and finally do what it takes to get the body and energy levels which will enable us to truly excel. It's up to you, but there is no way you would have bought a book entitled 'Turbo-charge Your Life' if you really thought all was OK with being just 'OK'. I don't want to be just 'OK' and neither do you. Don't settle for comparing yourself with others in order to gauge your own success; always strive to be the best you are capable of being in any situation. You may or may not be overweight or particularly lethargic, but I can guarantee *when* you do the 14-day programme you will find that you push yourself to *your* next level.

'Where's My BUT?'

You may feel I haven't addressed your 'but' (so to speak!), but to be fair we could be here for the next 100 pages trying to counter each one. Rarely do people have just the one 'but'. The minute you come up with a solution to a person's 'but', up pops another, and another. But … 'it's too cold', 'it's too hot', 'it's too wet', 'it's too dry', 'I'm working', 'I'm on holiday', 'the kids are on holiday', 'the kids are at school', 'it's a weekday', 'it's the weekend' … and so it goes on and on and on.

The general rule I have found is the more 'buts' a person comes up with, the bigger the *butt* they tend to have, and the more unfulfilled their life tends to be.

The reality is you can 'but' your way through the next God knows how many years, BUT if you do that, you'll never have the extraordinary life you deserve. You will also never feel the joy of what it's like to wake up every day in an energy-fuelled, slim, trim healthy body. You'll never experience what it's like to be the very best *you* can be, to live at your true potential every day. If you 'but' your way through life you'll always wonder what could have been.

It doesn't matter what decade of life you are in, how lethargic you are, how much money you have or don't have, how fat or thin you are, how many children you have, or whatever other 'but' you can come up with – *anyone* can change and get a body and daily life they are proud of.

'But My Story Is Different'

Unfortunately, some people have what they consider very big 'buts', buts which go way beyond 'I haven't got the time' or 'It's in my genes.' The sort of buts which they believe no amount of 'positive thinking' could possibly help with. Your particular story of why it's different or more difficult for you may well be moving, disturbing, painful and, on the surface, justified. However, if you want to move forwards, one thing must be clear:

We've **all** got a story –
get over it!

Everyone has had 'shit' happen to them, and virtually everyone you meet will tell you that they didn't have an idyllic childhood.

It is true that some people have worst pasts and stories than others, but it's all relative. After all, what one person perceives as bad or life-crippling can be just another day or even life-*enhancing* to others. Some people see their past as a valid reason for not having the life they want, whereas others use events of their past as a tool to drive them forwards to create a magnificent life.

Now I know that people's childhood experiences are a touchy subject, but as this is one of the major excuses for overeating, smoking, excessive drinking, not doing exercise and, for many, not getting a life, I feel the need to get real with this seemingly big 'but'.

If you had 'shit' happen to you as a kid, if you feel your childhood wasn't exactly a bed of roses, then you need to realize one thing – you're not alone. The sad reality of our world is that you don't need to pass any kind of exam to be a parent, and many people haven't got a clue. However, what has happened to you in the past doesn't *have* to dictate your future. It doesn't mean you have to drag it around with you for ever, and it doesn't mean you don't have a choice – because you *always* have a choice. You can either choose to allow past events to control your thoughts and your life every day; or you can use the experience as a motivation to drive you forwards. You can use it as a negative or a positive 'but'. You can say, 'But shit happened to me so what do you expect?' or, 'But sod it, I'm my own person now, I call the shots.'

I know many people who had extremely difficult childhood experiences. Some allow what happened to them all those years ago to justify their current behaviour and lack of life, while others who had exactly the same experiences thrive. Two sisters I know are a case in point. One sister has the attitude, 'They controlled my childhood but there's no way they're controlling me now', and has stopped smoking, barely drinks alcohol and eats well. She moved to Spain (she cycled there from England with a rucksack!), speaks Spanish better than some of the natives and runs her own successful business. Whereas the other sister, who had *exactly* the same upbringing, smokes and drinks heavily, lives off the state in a run-down flat, eats all the wrong foods and constantly bitches that life isn't fair and the world owes her a living.

On the surface, it's easy to blame her past for her current situation and behaviour; but if you look at her sister it doesn't wash. I'm not underplaying what people have gone through – some of the stories are nothing short of horrific – but what I'm saying is whatever horrors we experience, we can either become stronger, wiser and more driven because of them or we can drag them around with us like unwanted luggage and use them as our biggest 'but' at every possible opportunity.

It's *NOT* what *happens to you* but what you do with what happens to you that shapes your future.

It is so easy in this life to use past events, no matter what they are, as seemingly valid reasons for not having a compelling future. The reality is that it's not what happens to you, but what you do with what happens to you that counts.

Lance Armstrong's Story

Have you ever heard of a guy called Lance Armstrong? If you want to talk stories then let's have a very quick look at his. In 1995–96 he was one of the most precocious talents the world of cycling had ever seen and was on his way to becoming a cycling legend. On 2 October 1996, he was diagnosed with stage 4 testicular cancer. Testicular cancer is believed to be the easiest of all the cancers to cure; that is, unless it has reached stage 4 without detection. When the tests and x-rays came back it was even worse than they had feared; lesions had appeared on his lungs and brain and the doctors gave him at the very best a 40 per cent chance of survival. In his magnificent and heart-warming book, *It's Not About the Bike*, he wants people to know that going through chemotherapy isn't simply about losing hair, having a sickly pallor and wasting away. These are just side-effects of the treatment:

Chemo was a burning in my veins, a matter of being slowly eaten from the inside out by a destroying river of pollutants until I didn't have an eyelash left to bat. Chemo was a continuous cough, hacking up black chunks of mysterious, tar-like matter from deep inside my chest. Chemo was a constant, doubling-over need to go to the bathroom ... I felt like my veins were being scoured out ... I had no life other than chemo.

The race no longer became about the bike, but about who would kill who. Would the chemotherapy kill the disease before it killed Lance? Luckily for Lance, after months of hell, the chemotherapy killed the disease and not him. He was finally released from hospital in February 1997 in remission. He would have to wait a full year before he could safely say he was free of the disease in the long term.

At this stage, with everything he had been through, still in remission and with his body a shadow of its former athletic self, it would have been extremely easy for him to 'but' his way through the rest of his life without a flicker of protest from anyone. After all, he had beaten a horrific dose of cancer and just the mere fact he was alive proved to him and the world that he was a success. I don't think anyone would have said a word if he had decided to use this life event as a valid excuse for no longer seeking his dreams. Instead, he decided to do to what his mother had always taught him, to 'Make every obstacle an opportunity' and, boy, did he!

Once out of hospital he set about rebuilding his life. His passion was his bike, but now he could barely cycle up a small hill. This was simply an 'obstacle', which meant of course that it was an opportunity to show himself and the world what he was really made of. He slowly began training and setting himself seemingly impossible targets such as completing the Tour de France, for example. For those who don't know, I cannot emphasize enough that the Tour de France isn't just some bike race, it is the single most challenging bike race on the planet – simply finishing makes you superhuman. Just sixteen months after being released from hospital Lance finally had a chance to fulfil his dream – he entered the 1999 Tour de France. Everyone had written him off as a contender for the race and thought he was just the 'brave cancer victim' who was looking for some kind of sympathy cheer. Lance managed to cycle 2,500 km over the highest passes of the Alps and Pyrenees. Not only did he complete the race, which was perhaps one of the greatest ever sporting achievements given the extraordinary circumstances, but he won – and in the fastest ever time. Just to point out it wasn't a fluke, he came back the following year and did it again, and again the following year, and the year after that; and again in the following three years. To win just one Tour de France is superhuman; but to come back from death's door and win an unrivalled and record breaking seven back-to-back is nothing short of a miracle.

Lance Armstrong now says if he had a choice between winning the Tour de France or having cancer, he says he would take the cancer every time. Why? Because having cancer made him a better person and made him appreciate so many things he never did before. To Lance cancer was an obstacle which he turned into an incredible opportunity.

Whatever our stories we all have the same choice – and it is a choice. You can either choose to get the body and life of your dreams or you can choose to spend the rest of your life 'butting' and 'bitching' that you've been dealt a bad hand.

Michael Watson's Story

One Saturday night in September 1991 middleweight-boxing sensation Michael Watson stepped into the ring against Chris Eubank. It would be nearly a decade before he stepped anywhere again.

For 11 rounds Watson was winning the fight by a mile but just one almighty punch from Eubank in the 12th changed Michael's world for ever. The fight ended at 10.54 pm. and five minutes later Michael Watson started to die in the ring. A small lump of blood was forming on the surface of his brain causing severe pressure, and with every passing minute he moved closer and closer to death.

There is a 'golden hour' for people with head injuries and Michael was running deep into that precious hour by the time he was on his way to hospital. Unfortunately that hospital didn't have the facilities to do immediate brain surgery and valuable time was lost. The hospital did, however, put a tube down Michael's throat and blew oxygen into his lungs, without which he would have died. A brain scan revealed the clot and the next stage of the race to save his life was on. By the time he reached the next hospital the blood clot was the size of a saucer of milk and at that time there was nothing keeping his brain working. Michael ended up having six major brain operations and his life was on a knife-edge for many weeks, but miraculously he survived, just.

After nearly two years in hospital he finally went home, to a home and a life that was very different from the one he had left to go and fight Chris Eubank. There was no question that just surviving was a miracle in itself and Michael was incredibly optimistic when leaving, saying: 'I was a twenty-eight-year-old former professional boxer, and I couldn't walk, but to me the future looked bright.' But once home Michael soon realized that the first two years in hospital were simply the first round of what would be his biggest ever fight: the fight for a 'normal' life. He couldn't use his body, he needed help breathing with a ventilator, he couldn't communicate in the way he wished and he needed round-the-clock care. In his own words:

I felt like I was in prison ... I had words but I couldn't get them out fast enough. I wanted to walk and run, but my body would not let me.

He was told at one point he would certainly never walk or talk again and that real recovery was highly unlikely: he would probably be in a semi-vegetative state for the rest of his life.

Most people would accept the prognosis and just feel lucky to be alive, but not Michael Watson. Michael had other ideas, and vowed that one day he would not only get his speech back, but would walk again and lead as close to a normal life as possible. He knew the journey would be far from easy, and it wasn't, but he was willing to do whatever it took to achieve his dream. He wasn't willing to feel sorry for himself and tell the world, 'but there's nothing I can do about it', a 'but' which most people would have thought perfectly valid.

If doing what was necessary meant hours and hours of being in incredible pain while his helpers tried to manipulate his muscles to move, then so be it. If it meant having to refuse his mother's food in order to lose weight to make it easier on his helpers to move him, then that's what he did. Michael had a dream to walk and talk again and nothing was going to get in his way.

To cut an amazing story incredibly short, not only did Michael Watson walk again and regain much of his speech, but he even had the audacity to enter the 2003 London Flora Marathon! He, along with his neurosurgeon and now friend, Peter Hamlyn (the man who saved his life), thought it would be a good way to raise money for the British Brain and Spine Foundation. The only problem was that although he could walk a bit – which was nothing short of a miracle – he couldn't actually walk that far. In his moving book, *My Biggest Fight*, he says, 'All I had to do was add about twenty-six miles to the 385 yards I could walk at the time.'

Michael had just four months to somehow find a way to walk 26 miles further than he could walk. As he said, 'It was going to be an epic struggle, and one that would require every ounce of strength, determination and faith.' Even Peter Hamlyn thought it was madness, telling Michael that most marathon runners hit the wall after about 20 miles but that he would hit the wall after a hundred metres and would keep doing that until the end or (most likely) until he was forced to retire.

Just before the race Michael overheard Peter talking to journalists:

Michael has no business walking to the end of the road, never mind starting a marathon. If he achieves it, and it is a big 'if', it will be one of the greatest physical achievements the marathon has ever seen.

Everyone who was anyone came to cheer Michael through every mile. People were throwing money into buckets and he was joined by many, many friends, family and well-known people who would walk with him and keep him company. One such person was Alex Robinson, a twelve-year-old boy who was walking for the first time since being run over by a car in May 2002. Before Alex joined Michael in the marathon he couldn't walk at all. Michael had inspired him, which was one of the main reasons why Michael was doing the marathon:

I wanted to reach people like him who had given up hope of ever achieving their dreams. I had been told I would never walk or talk, and I had proved everybody wrong. I wanted other people to feel inspired to achieve the same thing.

It is amazing what people can achieve the minute they think it's possible. Before Roger Bannister broke the infamous four-minute-mile nobody thought it was possible for a human to run that fast. Yet the minute Roger proved it was possible another 37 people also broke the four-minute-mile in that same year. Alex Robinson was probably told that it wasn't possible for him to walk at that time, but the minute he saw it was possible for Michael, he decided to join him.

Michael saw so many heroic acts by the public along the way, all of which made him feel incredibly humble. There was even a homeless man under the bridge of the Embankment, who left his cardboard box and came over in his old clothes to give Michael the 70p that he had collected that day.

The mammoth and seemingly impossible task of actually completing the marathon was never going to be easy. Everyone knew that. By the end of day 2 Michael's feet were a mess. He had blisters on his toes and tremendous aches and pains; he even had to throw away his socks *en route* and replace them because they were so bloody. But Michael, in his own words, 'never quits' and on the second to last day he ignored the cut on his toe, his sore ankle and muscle strains; he ignored the fact that every step was pure agony and marched on.

When Michael Watson crossed the finish line the big clock above his head read **6 days, 2 hours, 27 minutes and 17 seconds**. In a marathon where Paula Radcliffe had set a record for the fastest ever time in the women's race, Michael too had set a new record – for the *slowest* marathon walk in history.

It seems ironic that just one year later the very able-bodied Paula Radcliffe would 'quit' the marathon *and* the 10,000 metres in the middle of each race at the 2004 Olympics in Athens because she was struggling. This is something Michael Watson would never even contemplate as he doesn't understand the word 'quit'. If it would have meant crawling to the end he would have done it. Paula battled hard to come back a few months later and win the New York Marathon, but it will take a few more non-quitting moments like that before she and other people forget. Paula used the pain of quitting to ensure that it will never happen to her again, and this is an amazing example of turning your obstacles into even greater opportunities.

Pain Is Temporary – Quitting Lasts Forever

Lance Armstrong and Michael Watson have one very common thread – they don't quit. In Lance Armstrong's follow-up book, *Every Second Counts*, he said that he would never have won even one Tour de France without the lesson of illness. He believes that his illness taught him an extremely valuable lesson: pain is temporary – quitting lasts for ever.

But Nothing!

For most of us, our daily lives are nowhere near as challenging as for people fighting cancer or trying to overcome a serious injury. Yet we still manage to bitch, complain, feel ungrateful and tell the world how things aren't fair because we have been dealt a bad hand. And we use the past as an excuse for our failings.

It's not the hand you are dealt, it's how you play it.

The only thing that sets the successes apart from the failures, the only thing that makes people either excel or falter, are the excuses. Some people see the obstacles in life – no matter how big – as opportunities; whereas people who continue not to achieve their dreams see them as impenetrable barriers.

Life isn't fair at times – that's true – but for most of us life is a blooming sight fairer than for most, especially when you consider that 50 per cent of the world's population lives on less than £1 a day! In fact, it is estimated that if you have some money in the bank, food in the cupboard for more than one day, a secure roof over your head and the ability to roam freely, then you are in the top 8 per cent of the world's population. If you also have your eyesight, the ability to hear and all your limbs in working order, you move up another per cent or two. Yet despite this, most people with such incredible opportunity in front of them look at the top *financial* 2 per cent and feel hard done by.

We would never have heard of Beethoven if he'd said, 'but I'm deaf' or Stevie Wonder if he'd spent his life saying, 'but I'm blind', or Will Smith if he'd said, 'but I'm black', or Billy Connolly or Oprah Winfrey if they'd allowed their awful childhoods to stop them living their dreams. We would never be on brink of a major breakthrough in stem-cell regeneration, which could pave the way for paraplegics to walk again, if Christopher Reeve had said, 'But I can't move or breathe by myself, so just pull the plug.'

I will repeat this point over and over again: it's not what happens to you, it's what you *do* with what happens to you that sets apart the success from the failures. It's what makes the difference between a life of 'FINE' and life of fulfilment.

So What's Your Story?

I was brought up in one of the worst parts of south-east London (and trust me, that's up against some pretty stiff competition!). I'm from a one-parent family with no brothers or sisters. We had very little money and I left school at 15. I was unemployed for years; I took drugs; and one of my closest friends died in his early 20s from heroin and alcohol abuse. I could go on and on and on but who cares and so what?

Everyone you meet will have a story and could easily use their 'unique' story of the past as a great excuse not to get a life today; to eat and drink rubbish and not live their dreams. This is great for the people who do this as they never have to take responsibility for their actions: it's always down to what happened to them in their past. It's always someone else's fault. How on earth can you expect to turbo-charge your life if you insist on letting the past drag you down? It's incredibly difficult to build up any sort of speed with all that dead weight hanging around your neck, and it's incredibly difficult to see where you're going if you keep staring in your rear-view mirror!

The only way to move forwards is to finally let go and allow yourself the opportunity to excel.

Whatever your 'but', whatever your story, I can guarantee it doesn't come close to that of the hundreds of thousands of people around the world who are coping with war and famine.

Unless you stop the nonsense excuses, the feeling hard done by, the blaming everything and everybody, you will never take your body, health and life to the next level. In other words, unless you lose *all* of your 'buts', you have no chance of permanently losing your butt.

You also have very little chance of losing or reshaping that butt unless you get off it!

Yes, the first point of call for reshaping your body and mind is finding a way to appreciate and use …

The Gift of Physical Movement

Get Moving

Exercise is not just for those looking to shift a few pounds; it benefits everyone who takes part. The problem, as we've seen, is that people will use just about any excuse in the book to avoid it, which is strange considering how flipping good we all feel afterwards. It is also odd considering that many people would literally give their right arm to have the ability to move.

Christopher Reeve was a man I admired greatly; he was without question a true Superman. In his second book, *Nothing Is Impossible*, he stated, 'I make sure I exercise every day as any hope of recovery is not possible without it.' What's amazing about that statement is that he was only 'hoping' he would reach his goals. His number-one goal, incidentally, was not to walk again, as many people thought, but to breathe unaided and to gain enough feeling to be able to hug his family. Yet despite the fact he had no idea if what he was doing would work, he spent nine years exercising (often in great pain) and eating well every day, praying it just might work, that it might aid his recovery in some way and help him have a better quality of life.

It must have frustrated him greatly to have lived in a country where over 60 per cent of the population is overweight or obese, and to know that the one thing that would *solve* their problem was the very thing he was dreaming of being able to do – MOVING THE BODY. It must have driven him crackers to hear people not only complaining about their weight but also bitching about *having* to exercise to make themselves better. These are people who have the incredible gift of physical movement and yet 'can't be bothered' to use it. These people also *know for certain* that their problem will be solved by moving their body.

Yes, it may be hard *initially* to get up and into the swing of exercise. We all know that after the first day you'll probably have more aches and pains than you've had in a long while; and those who have been through the experience will know that the following day is even worse. But pain is temporary; quitting lasts a lifetime. The effort or 'pain' is all relative and it's short-lived, but by not exercising you have to live that failure every day. People like Christopher Reeve are willing to do whatever it takes. They don't blame situations or other people; they just do whatever is necessary to achieve their goals, even if they are relying only on hope. The theme of the film *The Shawshank Redemption* was that without hope you have nothing. But if you are overweight, lethargic or both, you don't even need *hope*; your 'dis-ease' of the body will *certainly* be solved by eating well and *moving your body*. With dedication, you can easily change your body shape and boost your energy levels.

You and I are unbelievably lucky; we have the gift of movement. It is truly a wonderful gift which I think we often take for granted, and I just wouldn't dream of not using it. I also strongly believe that not to use it would be somewhat of an insult to those who have had the gift taken from them.

Still Me, Active You

I once listened to an audiobook version of Christopher Reeves' first book, *Still Me*. He recorded it a couple of years after the fall which left him a paraplegic. I remember putting the tape on at the start of my journey from Birmingham to London. It was so captivating that when I arrived at my destination I couldn't remember a thing about the journey. I pulled up outside my house, turned off the engine and continued listening to the tape. I have no idea how long I was there, but I didn't leave the car until I had listened to the entire tape.

Christopher talked and talked about his journey, and how he wanted to end it all and would have done if his wife hadn't said, 'You're still you' (hence the title *Still Me*). He described how tough it was to try to regain his speech and how he dreamt of the day he would be able to breathe by himself without the constant noise of a ventilation machine humming in his ear. Throughout the tape he sounded like a true Superman and you felt at stages he was accepting his condition and was learning to live with it as best he could. But then, at some point on the tape towards the end, he said that despite many things the best time of the day for him was when he went to sleep, for it was only when he was asleep that he could walk, run, play sports and be active. He would hate it if someone woke him up from a good dream, a dream where he was horse-riding or playing tennis. The dream world was often much better to what he had to wake up to.

You don't have to fall asleep to move; you don't have to try to direct your thoughts before you go to sleep in a desperate attempt to get into the physical world. You already have the gift of movement; it's a gift that many people dream of and it's a gift that will not only help to get you to the land of the slim and trim for certain, but will have a knock-on effect on every aspect of your life.

A good blast of exercise cleans your lymphatic system, flushes dead cells from the body, supplies oxygen to the body; and is an incredible stress reliever. The bottom line is it just makes you feel good! That good, clean, light feeling has a tremendous knock-on effect: it makes your mind sharper, your food taste better and takes your energy to a new level.

I once played tennis with a guy in the Canary Islands – Lance. He kicked my arse (or ass if you're from the US) 6–0, 6–0, 6–0. Now I'm not that good, but I'm a pretty decent player and can give anyone a good game – except this guy, clearly. It turned out he was 76 years of age and even had a replacement hip! When I asked him what his secret was he simply said, 'Whatever you do in life – KEEP MOVING' – and I have.

I remember when I was a child being able to get into all sorts of yoga positions; I could even do the Lotus position *while* walking on my knees (that's impressive, trust me). However, because I stopped, it would now take me many, many months of muscle manipulation and plenty of dedication to even hope to get in the same position again. The point is, if I'd carried on I would still be able to do it now and, like Lance, I would continue to do it way into my most mature years.

Movement is like a muscle. Use it or lose it!

If you were to, say, jump on a mini-trampoline every morning – as I often do with my main man Robbie Williams blasting on the stereo – there wouldn't be a point at which you couldn't do it any more, unless you got some kind of injury. If you did it every day, you wouldn't wake up one morning and not be able to bounce; your brain and body would be conditioned for physical movement, and it would be as automatic as breathing.

Finding the Right Exercise for You

There are a million ways to keep fit, and everyone's got their own idea of what's best. I love the mini-trampoline as it's not only fun – a key element to wanting to do exercise – but other than swimming, it's the only exercise that works every single muscle in the body with very little impact while giving a tremendous cardiovascular workout. I must point out here that not all mini-trampolines are made the same, and most can actually be jarring on the joints. I have a half-fold rebounder called The Pro-Bounce. The bounce you get is in a completely different league to the rebounders you may have tried. It is also the only mini-trampoline in the UK which you can fold in half, put in a carry case and transport to wherever you wish. It even has a support bar, which means no matter what your age, ability or size, you can still use it. I have two in my offices and a couple at home. Whenever I feel slightly sluggish, on goes Robbie and after a few minutes on the Pro-Bounce I'm back in business.

Even though we may all have our own exercise preferences, what's really best is to move and move and move. Many people think that if they go to the gym for one hour, three times a week it will make them slim and healthy, but there are 165 hours in a week. If you spend the other 162 hardly moving at all, welded to pieces of furniture, then clearly those three hours aren't enough.

Remember we are looking to turbo-charge your life, not pussyfoot around with half-hearted attempts, and that means stopping the excuses, getting up and really moving your body on a daily basis – and when I say move I mean MOVE.

Get Real

Those people who advise us to get more exercise by taking the stairs instead of the lift make me die. When I was fat, I would have needed to walk up and down the stairs of the Statue of Liberty twice a day to make any difference at all. For most overweight/unfit people, simply taking the stairs instead of the lift of their local NCP after parking the car makes about as much impact to their health and weight as 'One True Voice' had on the music industry (if you're thinking, 'One True who?', that proves my point!).

A recent book which accompanied the BBC TV show *Fat Nation* – which was meant to be a serious look at the obesity epidemic in this country and what can be done to help – had some amazing advice for physical activity which I just have to share.

One piece of advice blew my mind: 'Tips for couch potatoes – Don't sit on the sofa and change the TV channel using the remote control (which uses 1 calorie), get up to do it (using 3 calories).'

I really wish I were joking but someone actually sat down and wrote that piece of advice. First, who the blooming hell worked out that using the remote control uses 1 calorie and getting up uses 3? I think they make it up. If it were true, you wouldn't need to hit the gym; you could just sit and change channel 300 times an hour or simply move your thumb. Does anyone in their right mind really think that moving your thumb up and down 500 times burns 500 calories?

To be fair, though, this seems positively sane compared with the next gem I found in the book. Under the heading 'Our Fitness Expert Says' came the following: 'When you are watching TV as a family, all get up when the advertisements are on and do some activity. Rush off for a run around the garden, walk or run up and down the stairs, do some press-ups, or jump on the exercise bicycle. If the ad breaks are 2 or 3 minutes each, you can add quite a lot of physical activity to your evening. No stairs? Do knee lifts or walk or jog on the spot.'

Yes, you can add quite a lot of physical activity doing this … if you're mad as a goose that is! Jump up and down while the ads are on – are they having a laugh? Who the flipping hell would do that? And a fat lot of good this advice is coming from a programme on the BBC. 'Yes, I'll work out as soon as the ads come on' – you've got a long wait if you're watching the BBC. What possible use is running around your sofa for two minutes while the ads are on going to be for your weight and health? The only thing you'd lose by doing that is not your excess weight but your dignity and self-respect. Imagine popping around to someone's house and as soon as the ads came on the entire family got up and started doing press-ups – you'd run a mile (maybe that would work then, for you anyway).

Surely, better advice would be to exercise during the programme, not the adverts, or – and how's this for a bonkers idea – stop watching the blooming thing sometimes. Given that TV zaps so many of our precious hours and is one of the biggest causes of non-movement there is, I'd like to put forward a suggestion which was first made by a well-known TV show back in the late '70s/early '80s …

WHY DON'T YOU

switch off the television and go and **do something less boring instead?**

Do you remember the children's TV show called *Why Don't You?* If you do, you will remember just how effective the slogan was – *not!* Here we had a show that told us at the start to 'switch off the television and go and do something less boring instead' – so what did we do? Yep, we stayed exactly where we were and stared at the TV.

There is a great card from Larson which shows a family all sitting down watching a corner of the room with nothing there. The caption reads, 'Life before TV'! And when you look at the card it really does make you wonder what on earth we did before TV. I guess it was a strange time when people played games, read books, learnt about cultures and talked to each other; a time when you would make your own entertainment instead of sitting on furniture staring at more bits of furniture for hours on end – how bizarre!

A song in the 1990s had the chorus:

Television, the drug of the nation, breeding ignorance and feeding radiation, on television.

This may seem a little over the top, but methinks there's some truth in these words. Now I must point out that I'm not completely anti-TV. I don't know what I would do without my weekly dose of *Friends* and *Will and Grace,* or my bit of learning from a good BBC documentary; but there's no question that we are watching more TV now than at any time in history. Clearly, the history of TV isn't actually that old, but since Logie Baird invented the 'moving life in a box', the world and our health have certainly changed; and I for one believe the two are connected. I would even go as far as saying that the introduction of TV and the explosion of channels have been, in some cases, even *more* harmful to our health than many foods.

Widescreen Humans

A theory I've had for a long time is that it's not only the super-sizing of food portions that's making people fat, it's also the super-sizing of televisions. Haven't you noticed that people's waist sizes have increased in direct correlation to the increase in screen size? In the days of black-and-white TV, there were three channels to choose from, all of which began and ended at a certain time of day, and all TVs were 'normal' size, as were the majority of people.

Now we have 'super-duper plasma widescreen' with what appears to be a million different channels. At the same time, and by no coincidence I fear, we have 'super-duper widescreen' humans.

The average Briton now watches four hours of TV a day. Two of the most popular programmes are *EastEnders* and *Coronation Street*, both of which feature fictitious people living fictitious lives. Not that some people are aware of this you understand. There are many people who watch these 'soaps' who don't seem to be able to distinguish between fantasy and reality. When a character in *Coronation Street*, Deirdre, went to prison for some reason which escapes me now a national newspaper ran a front page with the headline 'FREE DEIRDRE'. If that wasn't nuts enough, given the many pieces of genuine news around the world that didn't make the front page, over 5000 people wrote in with donations to help free her. What scares the life out of me is that these people are legally allowed to vote! Most people clearly know that it's all fiction, but why make watching hours of fiction *your* reality?

We've even reached the stage where people spend hours watching late-night reality TV like *Big Brother*, sitting and staring at other people sleeping – has the world gone mad?

We've become focused on watching other people's lives instead of living our own.

Marilyn Manson

T*otal* V*egetable*

Curbing your TV and recreational computer time will, without a doubt, massively improve your mental and physical health. In the process it will give you back loads of precious time so many of us claim we don't have.

Television hypnotizes us for hours on end; it sucks our energy and robs of us our precious time, time which we can *never* get back again. It's true that we all like to 'veg out' in front of the TV from time to time, but we don't want to veg out so much that we turn into one. Perhaps that's why the expression which describes someone who sits in front of the TV and doesn't move from the settee for hours includes a vegetable – *potato* of the couch kind to be precise!

Not content with super-sizing our TVs, we have even super-sized the amenities with which we sit and watch them. There's a chair on the market at the time of writing called rather appropriately 'The La-Z-Boy'. This thing is almost like a sofa in itself. It is made of black leather, reclines almost like a bed and is made so that you never have to move. There are arms on both sides of the chair with lift-up compartments. These compartments are specifically designed to store your remote control, your TV guide and of course, your snacks. Under one of the arms to the side there is even a fridge for soft drinks and, naturally, beer. All it needs is a toilet and you'd never have to ever get out!

As well as specially designed furniture there is specially designed food to eat whilst watching the box – these are even known as TV dinners. Many snack foods are directly marketed for consumption with friends in front of the TV. These foods help to contribute to a lethargic state ideal for watching more TV.

WHATEVER *you* want to do *and* WHEREVER *you* want to go, *you* NEED mental *and* physical energy to MAKE it happen.

Box Culture

Many people now live in a box culture. We sit on box furniture, eating box 'food', whilst watching the box. Perhaps that's what they really mean by, 'it's time to think outside the box'. So why don't you, at times, do as the TV programme suggested and instead of aimlessly staring at junk TV for hours and hours, go switch off your television and do something less boring instead?

I'm being a little unfair as you are already way ahead of most of the box culture; you've actually got a book in your hand *and* you're reading it! That is much, much further than most.

In fairness not all people with weight, health and energy problems sit and stare at the TV for hours on end. Some do manage to pull themselves away from the box and go out ... to the cinema!

How many times have you thought I'll just sit down and watch a *little* TV only to find it has once again deprived you of yet another entire evening of your one and only precious life with its hypnotic gaze? Unless you plan your TV time and make strict TV rules for yourself, that seemingly innocent little box or flat screen on the wall will deprive you of years, yes *years* of your life.

In Britain we watch an average of 28 hours of TV every week.

Or to really hammer the point home, if we live until we're 70 we might have spent over 10 YEARS of our one and only life sitting on furniture watching more bits of furniture.

Imagine being given the gift of life and spending over 10 years of it sitting in a room staring at a box! Even if you halved your 'box' time you would free up 5 years of your life. Just think what you could do with those 5 or 10 years – write a book; learn a few languages; read hundreds of amazing books; learn how to play an instrument or two; take diving lessons; learn how to sing; travel the world; etc., etc., etc., etc., etc., etc., etc. ad infinitum.

Life is just too short and too precious to spend such a huge chunk of it staring aimlessly in front of a small box beaming flashing images at you.

If you are a 'soap head' and watch every episode of *EastEnders*, *Coronation Street* **and** *Emmerdale*, that will cost you a massive 2 years and 13 days, over a 60-year period and doesn't take into account the omnibus editions.

Internet Junkies

In some parts of the world, the problem of 'internet addiction' is now so bad that many teenagers are spending up to 14 hours a day playing interactive games. The winners become massive celebrities, taking on people in the 'finals' in huge stadiums with over 30,000 people watching the giant screens. This is clearly extreme internet use, but there's no question that, like TV, it's beginning to eat up precious hours, with many people checking their email 10 to 100 times a day.

Then you have 'normal' computer games, and boy have these come a long way since the two lines going up and down masquerading as tennis bats trying to hit a small square dot meant to resemble a ball.

There's nothing wrong with a *conscious* TV evening, a 'cinema day', checking emails or surfing the net. There are times on a cold, dreary English winter's day when I'll have a cinema day or rent about four movies and watch one after the other with a carpet picnic; and clearly I use the internet. What I'm talking about is when the TV or monitor just sucks you in and you end up sitting there watching rubbish or 'surfing' for hours and hours when you only intended to sit down for a few minutes.

As part of the 14-day Turbo-charge Your Life programme, you are not to watch more than two hours of TV *or* have more than two hours of 'recreational' computer time a day. If you use a computer at work, you have to take off any time spent looking at stuff which is not work-related – which for many would use their two hours alone! This means you need to start planning what you want to watch and exactly what you will be doing on the net, instead of aimlessly 'surfing'. You will be amazed at how much more time you have, and after a while the TV or computer may not even get a look in as you begin to expand your world with new hobbies and increased book reading.

What on Earth Did You Do?

Nobody really knows what happens to us when we leave this world, but my theory is we arrive on another plane. If I ever feel like I can't be bothered to do certain things, I imagine what it would be like to be greeted by the people on that plane. 'Hello, where have you just come from?' 'Earth.' 'Wow! What did you see, where did you go? Did you see the Grand Canyon? Did you learn to fly a plane? Did you visit a rainforest? Did you sample different foods from around the world? Did you swim with dolphins? Did you learn how to ski or snowboard? Did you lie in the Dead Sea? Did you learn different languages? Did you sail around the Greek Islands? How many people did you meet? Were you happy? Were you healthy? Did you watch the sun set in Hawaii? Did you, did you, did you?????'

Imagine being greeted with all that, being asked, 'What on Earth did you do?' and the only reply you could come up with was, 'Well, I went to work, drank some booze at weekends, sat down on some furniture most of the time watching other bits of furniture. Oh, but I can tell you everything that happened in *EastEnders*.'

This clearly is an exaggeration, but we are on Earth for such a short time, and there are so many things to see and do, it would be almost criminal not to expand your life and live, as opposed to merely surviving. When you think about it, we don't actually own anything; all we do is borrow it while we are on this plane. All we have are memories and experiences. Seventy per cent of people in the US don't even own a passport, and of the 30 per cent that do over 70 per cent of those have never used them!

So what on Earth are you doing? So what on Earth do you want to do?

We know that the gift of physical movement is our first point of call in making this a reality; but we also need the right fuel. And there is one thing you must do to make putting in that right fuel not only easy, but something you will do daily for the rest of your life …

Ditch the Diets

From the F Plan to Atkins, from the Hay Diet to the South Beach, from Weight Watchers to Slimming World – not a year, or even a month, goes by without the introduction of THE newest and best diet for one and all. There are also miracle 'fat' pills that promise 'amazing results', and creams, wraps, pumps, potions and patches that will 'help to melt away your body fat', 'reduce inches', or on the man side, 'pump up your muscles' or give you a 'guaranteed six pack'. And of course if all of that fails and you're really desperate, there's always the surgeon's knife!

The fact is, though, no matter what 'new' diet, patch, potion or pill comes out, the stats remain the same – diets have a 95 per cent failure rate.

And people know this *before* they start!

Despite this incredible failure rate, people still flock in their millions when the latest diet sensation hits the market. All it takes is for one slim, good-looking celebrity to say, 'I swear by this diet,' and before you know it every weekly women's mag has it on the front cover, tabloid TV shows are getting members of the public to try it out, and Amazon and WH Smith are quickly finding new space for this amazing diet phenomenon.

What few of us 'ordinary' people realize is that these celebrities are often constantly struggling with their weight and their food like the vast majority of people. In fact, nine times out of ten they are more hung up

DIETS have a 95 per cent failure RATE.

over their food intake and their bodies than Mr or Mrs Average. But because we think that all is well in celebrity land, people seem willing to follow just about anything they do, no matter how flipping bizarre it is.

One thing all diets have in common is that none of them deal with the *mental* side of dieting, which is precisely why the majority of them fail. Yes, some diets are doomed to disaster because of how little you are allowed to eat or the lack of good nutrition. However, the vast majority of diets fail, not because of some genuine physical deprivation, but solely due to a feeling of *mental* deprivation.

Dieting is Mental – in Every Sense of the Word

There is a wonderful sketch in an episode of *Men Behaving Badly* where Tony (the character played by Neil Morrissey) goes on a diet after being picked on by the other three main characters. We see Tony struggling with the diet, saying how difficult it is and how hungry he feels. His flat-mate, Gary (played by Martin Clunes), asks him how long he has been on the diet, to which Tony replies, 'One hour and thirteen minutes'!

This may be a little far-fetched, but not that far. Almost the minute people jump on a diet they immediately focus on the foods and drinks they can no longer have. In fact, most people start panicking about life without these foods and drinks days before they even start the diet. Clearly, this has nothing whatsoever to do with any genuine physical hunger, as they haven't even started the diet yet. It is *only* down to a *mental* feeling of deprivation. The truth is you can go on just about any diet you like, but unless the mental deprivation is eliminated, the diets will all feel pretty much the same.

A 'diet' only removes the foods causing the weight/health problem (and some don't even do that). They do nothing to deal with mental deprivation. This is crazy as it's *only* the perception of deprivation that makes the difference between being 'on a diet' and having *changed* your diet.

**If you do not feel mentally deprived you are *not* on a diet.
If you do – you are!**

What I want to get crystal clear is that being 'on a diet' is a way of thinking, not a way of eating. Yes, you change your way of eating at the same time, which is why people think it's always about the food, but the *feeling* of being 'on a diet' is a way of thinking.

**When you change your way of eating, you have *changed* your diet.
When you feel deprived because of it, you are *on* a diet.**

I remember once speaking to a few raw-fooders. These are people who only eat foods in their raw state. No, this doesn't mean they eat raw meat (although some do); it means they *only* eat things that haven't been cooked, such as fruits, vegetables, nuts and seeds. One of the guys I spoke with had been 'raw' for five years. I asked him if he ever craved cooked food, to which he replied, 'It's not easy being a raw-fooder. I love the smell of cooked food and I often miss it like crazy.' I asked if this feeling of deprivation was a recent thing, but he said he had found being a raw-fooder tough for pretty much the entire five years.

However, I spoke to another raw-fooder from the group who absolutely loved it. She had been 'raw' for six years and said she only very occasionally missed a bit of cooked food. She was grateful for how much energy she experienced daily and for having access to beautiful, nutritionally rich foods.

The *only* difference between the two raw-fooders was that one had *changed* their diet and one was still *on* a diet.

I want to make it clear that diet mentality is the *only* thing that causes people to struggle when they change what they eat and drink; it's not, as people believe, down to the food. To help you see this even more clearly, let me ask you a question. Have you ever felt really hungry during the day, and as you were about to go and get something to eat, something else stole your attention and you just forgot to eat? Some people may now be shouting, 'Not likely pal – I never forget to eat!' But I don't care who you are or how much you eat; I have yet to meet a single person this hasn't happened to at least once in their life. For most people it happens quite regularly, but *not* when they're on a diet. When people are *on* a diet, not only do they never forget one of their meals – ever – but food is on their mind *all* of the time, whether they're eating or not.

Think about it. When you are *on* a diet, you feel deprived when you are eating because it's not enough for your liking (or it's not the food you're used to). When you are not eating you feel as though you can't eat, and so again feel deprived. The point is, when on a diet you're always, to some degree, feeling deprived, and it's this *mental* feeling of deprivation that causes *all* of the 'struggle' people associate with dieting. As simple as it may sound, if you don't feel deprived you are not in a diet mentality, and the entire process of changing what you eat and drink becomes incredibly easy.

Why Feel Deprived?

This feeling of deprivation is madness. The 'struggle' is only caused by us, by the belief we are making some kind of genuine sacrifice. It's only caused by the bitching, moaning, moping and feeling sorry for ourselves; the feeling of being hard done by. But what on earth is there to feel deprived about? What sacrifices have really been made? How in blazes are we actually being 'hard done by'? We only changed what we ate and drank, and/or the amount we ate and drank, because the foods and drinks were causing us to feel like crap. They either clogged up our system making us bloated and lethargic, or they produced the most common symptom in the Western world today – TOO MUCH BODY FAT.

So why on earth do we moan about no longer having these disease-creating, life-zapping foods and drinks? I mean, it's not even as if we enjoy the entire experience of eating these rubbish foods anyway. Yes, we may look forward to what we believe they will be like and get excited *before* we eat; and yes, we may well enjoy the first and second hit of the drug-like food fix, but nine times out of ten we end up feeling bloated and thinking, 'Oh I wish I hadn't had that' or 'I wish I hadn't had *all* of that.'

So we often hate the feeling we get after eating these foods, and we also hate the physical results they create. Yet the minute we change (because we want the amazing results the new foods and new way of life will bring), we start complaining because we no longer have the very stuff that made us feel like rubbish in the first place! Is it me or does that just not make any common sense? When we are on a diet we spend most of our time moping around, missing something which, rationally, we hope we won't have. Please spend just a second thinking about how blooming bats that is!

The Can't Syndrome

This is where people get all worked up because they *believe* they 'can't' have certain foods or drinks and so go into a tantrum. I say 'believe' because, if you think about it, there is nothing actually stopping them from having whatever foods they want. What seems to have escaped them is that *they* are *choosing* to change their eating and lifestyle habits because they didn't like feeling the way they were. The acronym I use for can't in this situation is:

Constant And Never-ending Tantrum

And that's precisely what people put themselves through when using 'diet mentality' – a mental *tantrum*. A tantrum caused only by the *false* belief that they can no longer have certain foods or drinks, and a tantrum which just doesn't make any rational sense. It doesn't make sense to get annoyed and feel sorry for yourself because you don't have foods which you ideally don't even want. It doesn't make sense to envy people eating and drinking the rubbish that causes disease and over-weight. It doesn't make sense to tell yourself you can't have this or that when you can in fact have what the blooming hell you want. You *can* take heroin if you want. Nobody is actually stopping you (except the police); you just don't want to. The second we stop eating rubbish, we look at other people consuming the crap and start to envy them – but what the hell is there to envy? What we fail to see is that they are envying us. How many times have you stuffed yourself with a dessert after a big meal and at the end of it not only wished you hadn't had it, but also envied those who hadn't indulged?

The biggest mistake people make when they stop eating rubbish is that they rarely think 'Thank God I'm free of all that rubbish. At last I have the opportunity to get slim, trim and healthy.' All they do is complain and focus on what they think they can't have. I have a simple, yet highly effective, approach to stopping any 'cravings', or 'periods of adjustment' as I call them, during the 14-day programme *and beyond*. It's an approach which immediately stops the 'struggle' associated with 'diet mentality':

Either have whatever it is you believe you want and Shut Up
    or
Don't have it and Shut Up
... but whatever you do
SHUT UP!

Once again and for the final time: it's *only* the bitching and moaning that causes the problem; it's not some genuinely painful physical withdrawal from certain foods and drinks; and it's not a lack of nutrients to your cells (as your body will be getting the right fuel). It's just feeling sorry for yourself. If people were to just shut up and get on with it they would find it a doddle.

Focus on what you have the opportunity to have, not what you think you can't have.

We are unbelievably lucky to live in the Western world where nutritious foods are plentiful. We can buy an abundance of fresh fruits, vegetables, nuts, seeds, wholegrain complex carbohydrates and lean proteins just about anywhere. With the expansion of the internet, we don't even have to leave the house as many places will deliver all your nutrient needs to your door. Yet when people stop eating rubbish, all they can focus on is what they can't have.

The key to success on this programme is to start with a feeling of total gratitude – and the following story may just help you in that area.

Live Aid ... for Those Who Were Lucky

Do you remember 'Live Aid'? Most people not only remember it but remember exactly where they were when it took place. Do you remember the graphic pictures of starving Ethiopians with flies on their faces? It was these images which led one man – Bob Geldof – to decide that instead of simply watching like everyone else, he would get up and take massive action. Something had to be done and he knew the various governments around the world either didn't have the money to help, or had other more important agendas (like making bombs, for example). The result was a transatlantic concert with the biggest stars in the music industry taking part. Bob's actions raised an incredible amount of money and many lives were saved, but many weren't as lucky.

Now I don't know what you do for a living but spare a thought for this poor woman the next time you find it hard to make a decision at work. Claire Bertschinger was one of the Red Cross aid workers in Ethiopia at the time and her job was perhaps the most difficult I have ever come across or am likely to come across. There was a large area in the middle of a particular village surrounded by a wall, no higher than a couple of feet, where aid was distributed. Outside the wall there were many hundreds, if not thousands, of starving men, women and children and, because there wasn't enough food to go round, it was her job to have to walk along rows and rows of desperate starving people and to choose who would have food and who would be left. In other words: who would live and who would die. In her words: 'I feel terrible because it is sending them to a certain death. It is terrible; I can take just, just what we can.'

I, and I'm sure you, cannot possibly know how unbelievably hard and brave that task must have been.

One particular scene which was shown again when Michael Buerk revisited the area to mark the 20th anniversary of Live Aid, shows a beautiful young boy, sitting patiently in a row, waiting to see if Claire would choose him to step over the wall. The camera shows Claire walking along the row of starving men, women and children, picking various individuals who would get lucky. Claire couldn't pick the most malnourished as they might not survive even with the aid, making her task that much harder.

Often we didn't take the ones that were the worst, because they would die anyway. I didn't take them. I made sure I didn't take them because if I took them I would have kept them and that wasn't fair. I had to go up and down and pick the right ones and the right ones weren't necessarily the most malnourished, moribund ones because we knew they would be dead within twenty-four hours.

The camera then pans to the young boy's face. His face was aglow with such incredible hope. He had the biggest, brightest eyes, matched only by his grin. We then see the moment where Claire approaches where he is. His face gets even brighter, his smile even wider, as he looks up with unbelievable hope. The image after that I think will stay with me for ever. It shows the young boy losing that amazingly bright hopeful glow, placing his hands over his face and sinking his head into his chest. He hadn't been chosen.

I do not know if that boy lived or died, but what was incredible about the whole situation was the amount of dignity these people had in being chosen. The wall was just a couple of feet high and the thousands of starving people could have easily stormed it and tried to look out for number one. Instead they sat and awaited their fate with dignity. They accepted Claire's decision and continued to hope that perhaps the next day they might be chosen and perhaps if they were *lucky* they might get some rice and water. This incredible dignity was displayed on both sides of the wall. Those who were chosen, instead of yelling and screaming in joy, felt almost ashamed at the fact, especially given that those not chosen had a full view of those who could eat.

Bob Geldof sums it up by saying:

She (Claire) chose the ones who in effect would live and she could only choose a few, there was no protest from the others and the ones who were chosen for life in effect shamefacedly sat down on the ground inside the wall and put their head down.

We have no idea how unbelievably lucky and wealthy we really are. Unlike most people in the world, we have the opportunity to change what we eat, and we can choose the finest live foods, grains and proteins on the planet that will nourish every cell in our body and give us vibrant health.

When you jump on the Turbo-charge Your Life programme, be grateful for the foods and drinks you *can* have. Be grateful in the knowledge that these foods and freshly extracted juices will enable your body and mind to excel. Be grateful for the fact you can just nip to the shop and buy as much fresh produce as you choose.

You have an opportunity to bring foods, drinks and thoughts into your life which will help you truly excel. An opportunity to finally get the health and body you crave and *keep it!* In order to do this you need the right fuel, and as long as you *change* your diet and don't go *on* a diet, you have every opportunity to have the right fuel circulating in your body on a daily basis – without feeling deprived. But what exactly is the right fuel for the human body? With so many books, TV shows, magazines and DVDs all telling us different things, most people are now more confused than ever before – or so they say. I say this because we all have instinct, and although there is confusion over some issues on the nutritional front, we all pretty much know what's good and what's bad. To expand slightly on this, let's take a closer look at what exactly is …

The **RIGHT** fuel for the **human body**.

When I run stop-smoking sessions, rarely, if ever, do I get someone who thinks they know it all on that subject and most people are very willing to listen to what I have to say in order to gain freedom from that addiction. Equally, when I run an alcohol session, rarely do I encounter someone who thinks they're the world's leading expert on alcohol addiction. However, when it comes to the subject of food and health – everyone's an expert!

Everyone has an opinion about food and what is best for the human body. The subject is discussed somewhere in the country every second of each day. Office people converse about how many calories there are in each bite of a Caesar salad (without dressing of course!); people in supermarkets discuss food labels or debate that age-old dietary dilemma of which is better – butter or marg?; groups of friends chat over dinner about whether pasta is good or bad, or whether wheat was ever meant to be part of the human diet, or whether avocados are really fattening, or whether eating a grapefruit before each meal really helps you to lose weight, or whether the Atkins diet will destroy your kidneys, and so on and so forth.

This isn't exactly surprising when the subject of health, diet and fitness is discussed daily on just about every 'tabloid TV' show, almost every page of most magazines and every radio chat show, and newspapers are plastered with health-related 'shock' headlines such as 'ATKINS DIET IS NOT SAFE' (yes that made the front page!).

The crazy thing is if we were to get rid of most of what we believe to be true about what the best fuel for the human body from what we've 'headline' read and heard, and just keep to a touch of common-sense simplicity, we'd all be wiser and healthier.

Gut Feeling

The reality is we *are all* experts in the field of nutrition, in the same way that every single wild animal on the planet is an expert on their particular nutritional needs. The only difference between us and them is they don't go around discussing what they *think* is best based on some 'new' research from Harvard. They simply eat and drink what they *instinctively know* to be the best fuel for them; they use their 'gut feeling'. And if we cut through all the rubbish info about health we're bombarded with on a daily basis and go with our gut feeling instead, we all, to some degree at least, know what's best. Yes, there may be some confusion about certain parts of the nutritional jigsaw puzzle – such as what's the best form of carbohydrate – but fundamentally, on a gut level, we know what's right and what's wrong.

I mean, it hardly takes a NASA scientist to figure out that fast-food burgers, fries and a heavily sugared drink is bad for us, and that fresh, ripe fruits and vegetables, which are teeming with colour and nutritional vibrancy, are unbelievably good for us. It also doesn't require a PhD from Oxford University to know that fresh fish and some lean meats aren't the worst food choice you can make, or that eating a large plate of bread and butter isn't the best.

All we need to do is trust our own instincts and eat the *vast majority* of foods which our 'gut' tells us is good for us when we feel *genuinely* physically hungry.

If we just did that – and as long as we weren't on a 'diet mentality' – our food and weight problems would cease to be, and we would never have to worry about them again. In other words, we would be free from 'fad' diets and able to live a life in which we can eat freely – something the vast majority of people *never* achieve.

In case of any confusion about true gut feeling and about what's really best for the human body – and to finally lay a lot of nutritional codswallop to rest – I have devised The Six Essential Dietary Needs (page 140) and The Seven Deadly Dietary Sins (page 106). Both make it very easy to see what to eat, what not to eat and how much to eat.

After the 14-day Turbo-charge Your Life programme, which contains some specific dietary guidelines, *staying* on the healthy-eating track is very easy. The *vast* majority – about 70 to 80 per cent – of what you eat and drink should come from natural foods and drinks with a high water content found in The Six Essential Dietary Needs (such as fruits and veg). About 20 to 30 per cent should come from others foods that contain some of the essential six (such as fish, grains, nuts, seeds, meat). Very little, if any, should come from The Seven Deadly Dietary Sins. As long as you eat *only* when you are genuinely physically hungry, eat slowly and stop eating just before you are uncomfortably full, you are done and dusted. It's that simple!

This is why it is absolutely imperative that you read *all* of The Six Essential Dietary Needs and *all* of The Seven Deadly Dietary Sins. To miss them would be a fundamental mistake as without *all* of the necessary information you will not be armed with *all* of the tools you need to excel on a mental *and* physical level.

It's worth knowing at this juncture that *all* fruits and vegetables contain, to some degree, *every single one* of the six essential dietary needs. All fruits and veg are incredibly high in water too, designed to transport the live nutrients they contain quickly and efficiently to the many cells of the body. The high water content is also designed to help flush rubbish from the system. Getting a good supply of high-water-content, nutrient-packed foods and drinks is the single most important thing you need on a dietary level.

However, because of the amount of processed, water-less, lifeless food we have consumed for God knows how many years, our often tired, weak and blocked systems can have great difficulty extracting the maximum water-rich nutrition from the fibres of these amazing foods. For many people, this means that the water-rich nutrients contained in even the small amount of fruits and veg they *may* be eating aren't actually hitting the mark. It's not just about how many nutrients you are eating, but how many are actually getting through to where they are most needed.

With this in mind, I want to show you a truly amazing way for your body to gain the *maximum* nutrient content from fruits and vegetables. And it's the water-rich nutrient content that ultimately feeds the body and can only be described as …

Liquid Engineering
for Your Body

It's the juice of the fibre that feeds you.

Jay Korditch

The human body was designed specifically with liquid fuel in mind. It's no coincidence that every single plant food designed for the human body is over 70 per cent liquid. This life-giving fluid found in *every* single fruit and vegetable is nutritionally way beyond anything humans can manufacture. There simply isn't a pill, potion or supplement that comes even close to the power of this incredible liquid fuel.

Over the years, however, we have eaten fewer and fewer of these foods. This has blocked and weakened our digestive systems, making it difficult for the body to extract the powerful liquid fuel from the fibres of food. The amount of water-rich live foods – raw fruits and vegetables – in the average UK diet is only 5 per cent, when it should be at 70 to 80 per cent!

When it comes to optimum nutrition, the body's ability to extract the juice from the fibres of natural food is of paramount importance.

Clearly we need fibre, but you must understand that fibre does not feed you: it's the *juice* of the fibre that feeds you. The fibre is there as an aid to keep things moving (if you know what I mean) and as a neat tool to help transport liquid fuel in a solid form.

The key is to find a way to help our weakened, battered and blocked digestive systems extract as much of that life-giving juice as possible. After all, what's the point in finally getting around to eating a load of fruit and veg only to discover that just a tiny fraction of the nutrient-loaded fluid is actually getting to where it's desperately needed? There is only one thing to do:

Get Juicing!

Dr Norman Walker was perhaps the most famous advocate of freshly extracted fruit and vegetable juices. He was 113 when he died peacefully in his sleep, disease-free. He worked right up until the day he passed away and dedicated his life to teaching others how to gain optimum nutrition from nature's finest foods. He strongly believed that juicing was the best and easiest way to get live nutrients flowing in the bloodstream.

I know that if I do not drink a sufficient quantity of fresh raw vegetable juices every day then, as likely as not, my full quota of nourishment enzymes is missing from my body.

Dr Norman Walker

In case you are wondering what an enzyme is, let me put it simply – enzymes are life. Enzymes are as important to our food as vitamins, minerals, fats, carbohydrates, proteins and water. Without the presence of enzymes in the food, the body has to literally rob its own bank account. It is worth knowing that all heavily processed foods – foods which take up about 95 per cent of supermarket shelves – are void of enzymes; in other words they contain no 'plant life force'. This means that every time you have a burger, bun, pizza, ready meal, or anything else that comes in a packet, tin or can, your body has to dip into its own enzyme resources to make up the shortfall.

You lose enzymes through stress, alcohol and processed foods. You can't get them back from Diet Coke, hot dogs or coffee. You can only replace them with raw, whole foods – including juices.

Dr A Rosenberger

In other words, once your enzymes are spent – so are you!

Let Juice Be Thy Medicine

The healing power of the fluid contained within raw fruits and vegetables isn't a new discovery. Hippocrates, known as the 'father of medicine', is perhaps most widely remembered for his catchphrase, 'let food be thy medicine', and you can bet your bottom dollar that he wasn't referring to burger and fries! When he spoke of foods which should be 'both thy food and thy medicine' he was referring *only* to natural foods containing the 'elixir of life'. When he said 'let food be thy medicine', what he really meant was 'let the *juice* of the food be thy medicine'.

Freshly extracted vegetable juices have been used widely to treat and help prevent just about every disease known to humankind. Max Gerson MD found that when he put his 50 cancer patients on a juice-therapy regime, *all* recovered through his natural, 'gentle' treatment. I'm not saying that juicing can cure cancer, or that Gerson therapy will work for everyone; I'm just pointing out that this particular juice experiment had truly remarkable results. (For further details of this case study see Gerson's book *A Cancer Therapy: Results of Fifty Cases*.)

Max Gerson wasn't the only one to use freshly extracted juices to feed life back into the cells and to treat and *prevent* disease. The late Dr Bircher-Benner, founder of the famous Bircher-Benner clinic which also focuses on the power of raw juice, said 'There is nothing more therapeutic on earth than green juice.' Another great juicing mentor of mine is Jay Kordich. He has been teaching the healing and health benefits of freshly extracted fruit and vegetable juices for many years, and is well known for his statement 'All life on earth emanates from the green of the plant.'

Dr Norman Walker was convinced that of all the ways to treat and *prevent* disease, having a couple of glasses of freshly extracted vegetable juice daily, as well as keeping the system free of junk, was the most effective by far.

Ross Mansergh is one man who would completely agree with Dr Walker. He is 100 per cent convinced that the power of freshly extracted fruit and vegetable juice completely cured his cancer. When he was diagnosed, he chose to juice his way to health instead of using conventional medical treatment. He juiced his way through 75 pounds of carrots, 60 apples, six red cabbages and 25 pounds of leeks *every week*. In his own words: 'The best way to beat cancer is not to poison the body further, but by feeding it the right nutrients.'

The best way to beat cancer is not to poison the body further, but by feeding it the right nutrients.

Clearly there are a million and one different factors to a disease like cancer, and there is no question that in many cases medical intervention needs to play a part. But cases like that of Ross Mansergh and the 50 cancer patients treated by Max Gerson show that Nature's finest liquid fuel can weave its magic.

Many people in the medical profession pour scorn on 'juice therapy', especially methods such as Gerson's. They often get very angry with what they describe as 'alternative' therapies such as juicing. However, what I want to make crystal clear is that the life-giving juice trapped in the fibres of Nature's finest foods is not an 'alternative'; it's what the body craves and needs to heal itself. The term 'alternative' can often be more applicable to conventional drugs.

We have even reached the stage where it is illegal to advertise the fact that any food can help with a disease. The supermarket chain Asda was fined heavily in 2004 for advertising that mangos can help cancer, and had to withdraw the claim immediately. Yet the humble mango is rich in a known anti-cancer agent – beta-carotene – as well as vitamin C, many B vitamins, calcium, magnesium and potassium. On top of this, like all fruits and vegetables, it is loaded with antioxidants, which help keep the body free from disease.

If Hippocrates were alive today and wanted to open an organic fruit and veg shop with his slogan 'let food be thy medicine', he would probably be fined or closed down.

If I were a conspiracy theorist, I would say that the drug companies, along with the government, have some kind of vested interest in giving the impression that Nature's food cannot heal or prevent disease, and that drugs are the only way; but I'm not, so I won't!

At this stage I must point out that I'm not one of those people who believes that any disease can be cured with freshly extracted juice, or any complementary therapy for that matter. Nor am I one of those people who thinks you should never use medical drugs; because *at times* they are absolutely essential. But I have a very strong belief that the life-giving juice contained in Nature's water-rich foods is the finest fuel for the human body and is the best way to prevent and help treat disease. If a disease has progressed too far then, yes, medical intervention needs to come into play, but it needs to do so along with the right fuel.

This is why it blows my mind when you see the food dished out in hospitals. You would think that if there's any place guaranteed to supply the best fuel to heal the body it would be a hospital. Instead, we not only have trays of food that would make any economy airline's offerings look like the world's finest cuisine, but we even have fast-food outlets in the grounds of some hospitals.

And That's Magic!

Never underestimate the nourishing and healing power of what Nature has provided in the liquid of raw fruits and vegetables. If it can help in some cases of a severe disease like cancer, then imagine the kind of magic it can weave on a tired, lethargic and/or overweight body.

Magic, I guess, is the apt word for what happens when you begin to nourish your body with freshly extracted juice on a daily basis, along with the absence of The Seven Deadly Dietary Sins (page 106). Your hair starts to shine; your eyes start to sparkle; your skin begins to glow; your energy explodes; and if you need to lose weight – it just falls off! In fact, if you were to put yourself on a short-term plan of consuming *only* freshly extracted vegetable and fruit juices, you would lose 1 to 2 lb every two to three days. Notice I didn't say a juice 'fast' but a 'plan'. A fast is where no food at all comes into the body. What must be clear is that the juice contained within the fibres of raw fruits and vegetables *is* food – liquid food that flows through the body and feeds the cells with incredible ease.

When people come to our one-week mind and body juice retreat, it's amazing but true that they just don't feel that hungry after the first couple of days. During the week we consume *nothing* but freshly extracted organic vegetable and fruit juices. We swim in the sea and do yoga and meditation. This is because, for once, the body is getting the water-rich fuel it craves *on a cellular level*. What's also very noticeable after the week is the incredible weight loss experienced by those needing to lose weight – an average of 6 to 8 lb. People who go on the maximum juice-only resort plan, which runs for three weeks (and does include *some* apples and avocados for fibre), experience an average weight loss of 12 to 16 lb. They also require much less sleep, and their energy levels are through the roof compared with what they were before. Many, in just that short space of time, also become clear of all kinds of ailments which had been with them for years, such as IBS.

Living on nothing but freshly extracted juice can be seen as pretty extreme, but as long as you're not on diet mentality, it's a breeze. Juice alone is not what the Turbo-charge Your Life programme is about, as you will see, but juicing clearly does play a part. You will be making freshly extracted juice every day on the plan. I can guarantee that after you see the results, you and your juicer will never be parted.

Freshly extracted juice is not just an excellent healing aid; it is the best health-insurance policy you can invest in. You need to understand that it's much, much, much easier to prevent disease than it ever is to try to cure it. When you make a juice, you aren't simply making a delicious drink; you are creating the ultimate health tonic packed with vitamins, minerals, the *right* sugars, the *right* fats, the *right* salts, water, and amino acids (the building blocks for protein).

All in Good Taste

I'm not exaggerating when I say that freshly extracted juice is liquid gold for the body and mind. Every time you have a glass you will start to feel the 'live' goodness flowing through your system within minutes. It is hard to know where to stop when singing the praises of freshly extracted juices; they really are that good. And the taste of juices you make at home is in a completely different league to the 'enzyme-less' versions you see in bottles, cartons and cans in shops.

If you think you've tasted pineapple juice because you've had some from a bottle, you are in for one hell of a treat when you make it yourself.

It's rich, creamy and produces a 'head' almost akin to a Guinness. Even vegetable juice, when made the right way, tastes nothing short of beautiful.

The problem is most people have never tasted the rich, creamy, sweet liquid sunshine you get from fresh, just-juiced vegetables. The only vegetable juice most people have tried is carrot, and again it's usually the heat-treated version in a bottle and not the beautiful stuff you get when you make it yourself. When it comes to vegetable juices, it's the idea more than anything else which is off-putting. Most, I will admit, do sound, well, awful! On top of that, people often don't know what they're doing. They get hold of a juicer, read that spinach and cucumber juice is good for you, make it, take a sip, spit it out – and the juicer never sees daylight again. Even with my taste buds, if I had just spinach and cucumber juice I'd also spit it out because, on the taste front, it sucks! But if you simply add a little freshly extracted apple and pineapple juice, a pinch of ginger and a splash of lime, you get all of the life-giving goodness from the freshly extracted green juices without any of the awful taste. In fact, all you taste is a rich, sweet and creamy drink.

Vegetable juices are really what freshly extracted juice is all about. I tend to eat my fruit and *drink* my vegetables. Don't get me wrong, I also eat plenty of vegetables; but whenever I make a juice you can guarantee that things like spinach, broccoli, celery and cucumber will almost always get a look in – plus of course some apple, pineapple or carrot to help sweeten. It was juicing vegetables, not fruits, which got me into juicing in the first place. At that time I didn't eat anything remotely healthy. I wouldn't touch a piece of broccoli with a bargepole. But ever since I tasted my very first rich, sweet and creamy vegetable juice – which was celery, cucumber, apple and spinach – I was hooked. I had found a way of getting vegetables into my body without having to eat them – that was good enough for me! Since then, I have changed many aspects of my eating and now love vegetables like broccoli.

But even though I love *eating* vegetables, you cannot beat the power of 'raw' nutrition in a liquid form. Whenever you start to apply heat to vegetables you immediately begin to destroy the enzyme 'life' content within.

This doesn't mean that steamed vegetables aren't good, but 'live' nutrition in a liquid form has the highest enzyme content.

And because the machine has extracted the juice, you can be guaranteed that every drop of the liquid engineering reaches parts of your body that vegetables you eat often cannot. Again, this doesn't mean you shouldn't also eat freshly steamed vegetables as we need the fibre, and there are no foods richer in the right kind of fibre for our systems than fruits and vegetables. It just means raw juice also needs to play a part. And it's the raw *green* juice you're looking for to make the biggest difference.

Green vegetables contain a substance called chlorophyll. The famous research scientist, E Bircher, described chlorophyll as 'concentrated sunshine', and in a way that's precisely what it is – sunlight energy trapped within the fibres of the plant. This liquid sunshine improves the functioning of the heart, the vascular system, the intestines, the uterus and the lungs; it cleans and detoxifies the blood and liver, helps to strengthen the immune system and reduces high blood pressure – and that's just what is known. This is why you will see that vegetable juices feature quite heavily on the 14-day plan. Don't knock them until you've tried them.

Even if vegetable juices did taste disgusting, given the amazing changes they have brought me personally in terms of weight loss, energy and overall health, I would just hold my nose and pour the stuff down. Fortunately, they do taste incredible, and I now adore even the ones I initially thought a bit weird.

Why Juicing Provides Raw Energy

To understand even further why juicing is so powerful, we need to look at the process of digestion in a bit more detail. One of the most energy-consuming processes the human body undertakes is the digestion, assimilation and elimination of food; or to be more accurate, the digestion, assimilation and elimination of the *wrong* kinds of foods. In fact, you could even argue that the process of trying to turn inadequate food into usable body fuel and eliminate the waste is *the* most energy-zapping process the body can go through. If in doubt, let me ask you a couple of questions:

1 Have you ever felt tired after a meal consisting of a load of cooked and processed food?
2 Have you ever felt tired after eating a bunch of grapes?

All of Nature's foods have been more or less pre-digested by the plant, and all contain digestive enzymes, leaving the body very little work to do.

This is why you can eat as many oranges as you like but not feel sleepy, yet a large bowl of pasta can have you in 'nod nod' land before you can say *linguine al pesto*. It's worth knowing that when you overeat denatured food to the point of falling asleep immediately afterwards, you aren't so much in 'nod nod' land but in a coma! As scary as this may sound, what's actually happening when you 'doze off' after stuffing yourself with stodge is that the body doesn't have enough energy to keep you alive and awake at the same time.

In order for the body to try and turn this heap of semi-dead 'food' into some sort of usable body fuel *and* extract the wastes it creates, it needs energy – and lots of it. To do this, the body will shut down all 'departments' which aren't required for the job in hand. This is why eyesight, hearing and consciousness are usually the first to go – in that way all physical movement (apart from breathing) will also cease. This means the body can then use all its available resources trying to deal with the mass of denatured, often water-less, food that has just piled in. The entire process of digestion, assimilation and elimination can take hours, days, months, and even years. In fact, in many cases the process *never* fully happens.

We are Full of Shit – Literally!

You have over 30 feet of intestinal tract, designed with the right kinds of food in mind. Even from pictures, it's hard to get an idea of just how many twists and pockets there are in the small and large intestines. It is in these 'pockets' where you will find some of the hard-to-digest food leftovers which were eaten days, months and even *years* ago.

When you consume denatured foods on a *daily* basis, the body cannot always deal efficiently with them, and bits are often left undigested in the colon. In fact, many people have clogged their systems so much over the years that their colon may have a build-up of waste matter which has gradually hardened and stuck to the walls, reducing a 6 cm-wide tunnel to one as narrow as just a few millimetres. So the situation can sometimes be like trying to shove a watermelon through a Polo mint!

This means that our built-in 'juice extractor' – the one we have all owned since birth, designed to pull the juice from the fibres of Nature's foods in order to feed us – can no longer be as effective. This is why juicing is so flipping wonderful. When you put raw fruits and vegetables through a man-made juice extractor, you've effectively done the body's work for it. You have skipped the digestive process, a process which can take more energy than anything else, and have effectively furnished your cells with raw, live nutrients in the fastest possible way.

Weight off Your Mind

All of this helps to free up energy in the body, which it can then use to start breaking down the old, rotten food stuck in pockets and to the walls of the colon. This gradually leaves you feeling much lighter, physically and mentally. Even slim people will feel the benefits as it's not just overweight people who get bloated and full of shit.

With the risk of getting crude again, have you ever heard people coming out of the toilet saying, 'Oh, that's a weight off my mind'? Although it's not exactly the most pleasant thing someone can say, it is none the less very accurate. If your colon is full, it affects how you feel not only physically but also mentally. This is why if someone 'cannot go', it will massively affect their mood; when they do finally get some release they feel like a different person. This is clear when someone is very constipated, but what most people don't realize is that they are, to some degree, in a *constant* state of *constipation*. You simply cannot have a load of shit stuck in pockets and to the walls of your colon without it affecting your mind. In order to turbo-charge any aspect of your life you need to be mentally focused on what you're doing, and you will always be more mentally clear if you are also physically clear.

If you put juice in your body today, you'll have a much better tomorrow.
Jack La Lanne

Jack La Lanne is certainly a man who is pretty clear on every level. Have you heard of him? Well, if you have ever surfed the satellite TV channels late at night you may have seen him selling his juicer. I may not be a big fan of the juicer itself, but the man – well, what can I say. He is an 89-year-old food, health, fitness and juicing guru. In the States he is known as the Godfather of Fitness, and, to be fair, for bloody good reasons. When he was 60 he pulled a 100 lb boat across the San Antonio River with his hands cuffed and legs shackled! He apparently does the same thing every decade and adds *more* weight every time. He, even more so than Dr Walker, is completely convinced that juicing is the key to supreme health, vitality and physical vibrancy. He apparently wakes up at 5.30 a.m. every morning and works out for two hours every day. That may be your idea of hell, but whether you would *want* to or not, wouldn't it be nice to know you *could*, especially at 89 years of age?

A friend of mine was competing in an Olympic distance triathlon early one Sunday morning. I had no idea he was taking part until the day before. In my wisdom I thought I'd also have a bash. He explained that he was trained for it and that it would be foolish to take part. Being my foolish self, I phoned the organizers, borrowed a wet suit and a bike and was up at 4 a.m. making the drive to compete in (well, try and finish) the Olympic distance triathlon. We had to swim, in what I can only describe as a cold and dirty lake (we couldn't see anything through our goggles) for 1500 metres (a metric mile) then jump on a bike and cycle in very suspect weather for 50 km and then, as if that wasn't enough, run for 10 km!

I finished in under two and half hours. This isn't exactly an amazing time to say the least, but I was far from last in the pack. The reason for telling this story is not to show off, but to show that even if you have no intention of ever doing anything as crackers as an Olympic distance open-water swim triathlon, it is bloody wonderful knowing that with one day's notice you can have the physical and mental resources to join in if needed. Although my friend said I hadn't trained, in a way I was training every day. I make a point of working out on a daily basis, getting juiced and eating well.

It's not about completing a triathlon or marathon – it's about having the physical and mental vibrancy to tackle any of life's challenges with much greater ease.

It's about being able to live whenever you want to. It's about waking up and actually feeling awake. And one of the best ways to guarantee that your cells are getting a daily supply of what they need to thrive is with the power of raw freshly extracted juice.

And for those who say, 'Oh but juicing is a hassle and you have to clean the machine' please once again re-read that particular 'but' in

'The But Syndrome' if you've forgotten it and make a big point of always remembering you are doing this for *you*. You will reap the benefits and it's *your* life that will excel. So, as is the theme of the book, stop looking for buts, stop looking for excuses and just, for once, get on with it.

You Cannot Live on Juice Alone

As powerful as juicing is, you need to understand that you cannot, and should not, live on *just* juice. Juicing is a neat catalyst to the land of the slim, trim and healthy, and it's without question the single best health insurance you and your family will ever invest in. However, you must realize that juicing is just *one* aspect of the programme. Equally as important are mental attitude, physical exercise and – eating.

I love juice, but I also love to eat. After a long day there are few things as satisfying as ending genuine hunger with some beautiful nutrient-packed food.

I try to make sure that the foods I choose contain some or all of the elements that make up The Six Essential Dietary Needs and very few, if any, of The Seven Deadly Dietary Sins.

I have mentioned that everyone and their mother has an opinion of what's good and what's bad. I have also mentioned that, above all else, your 'gut feeling' is usually correct. However, due to years of misinformation, it can be hard to know if it's your gut feeling telling you whether a food is good or bad or what you've been taught. During the next two sections of this book – The Seven Sins and The Six Needs – I have presented some facts and some common-sense thinking about what's best for the human body. Please do not make the mistake of skipping these sections …

The Seven Deadly Dietary Sins

'Deadly' may sound somewhat over the top, but as the following dietary sins contribute heavily towards hundreds of thousands of premature deaths every year in the UK alone, I don't think the word is out of place. It is worth knowing that the wrong kinds of foods – foods high in refined salt, fat and sugar – contribute to more disease and premature deaths than *all* illegal drugs combined!

Eliminating all seven deadly dietary sins from the diet may be asking too much. Given that they're hidden in almost every convenience food we consume, it may even be an impossibility. But cutting down on them *drastically* and swapping them for an abundance of foods from the Six Essential Dietary Needs (page 140) will make a significant difference to your body shape, energy levels and overall health.

Refined Sugar Refined Fats
Alcohol **Artificial Sweeteners** Caffeine
Salt Dairy Products ***Refined Sugar***
Refined Fats Alcohol Artificial Sweeteners
Caffeine Salt *Dairy Products* Refined
Sugar REFINED FATS Alcohol
Artificial Sweeteners **Caffeine** Salt Dairy
Products Refined Sugar Refined
Fats ***Alcohol*** Artificial Sweeteners **Caffeine**
Salt Dairy Products *Refined Sugar*
Refined Fats Alcohol **Artificial Sweeteners**
Caffeine Salt Dairy Products
Refined Sugar **Refined Fats** ALCOHOL
Artificial Sweeteners **Caffeine Salt** Dairy
Products **Refined Sugar** Artificial Sweeteners

1. **Refined Sugar:** the Cocaine of the Food World

I have no desire to pussyfoot around this one. White refined sugar is without question more dangerous to our health than any other food product. Sugar is not only becoming the new tobacco in terms of addiction, but it now contributes to *more* degenerative disease and premature deaths than tobacco.

It took many, many years for the tobacco industry to admit its product was highly addictive and dangerous, and I guarantee it will take even longer before we see the makers of refined sugar and carbohydrates doing the same. Some tobacco companies *still* refuse to accept their product is harmful and addictive, so I should imagine we have at least 50 years before the full truth about refined sugar is out.

When I mention sugar, I'm not just talking about the granulated stuff you put into your tea and coffee. I'm also talking about *all* refined carbohydrates, such as bread, pasta and flour, as once eaten they are quickly converted into glucose (sugar) in the body. Every time you eat a cream bun, a croissant, a biscuit, a white-bread sandwich or a muffin, you are eating SUGAR! You are also eating pure sugar when you see any of these descriptions on food labels:

- Corn syrup
- Dextrin
- Dextrose
- Fructose
- Fructose syrup
- Invert syrup
- Maltose
- Sucrose
- Treacle
- Molasses
- Palm sugar
- Golden syrup
- Maple syrup

I'll buy a huge piece of meat, cook it up for dinner, and then right before it's done, I'll break down and have what I wanted for dinner in the first place – bread and jam ... all I ever really want is SUGAR. [my emphasis]

Andy Warhol, *New York Magazine*, 31 March 1975

White refined sugar and carbohydrates are addictive poisons. That may sound over-the-top, but if we went back 25 years or so and suggested such a thing about tobacco, that would also have been seen as somewhat over-the-top. The highly possible nightmare side-effects of regular refined sugar consumption are nothing new. Many years ago, William Duffy, bestselling author of *Sugar Blues*, wrote the following about sugar:

Here is something more intoxicating than beer or wine and more potent than many drugs and potions then known to man ... it was a brain boggler. It could cause the human body and brain to run the gamut in no time at all from exhaustion to hallucination.

And Duffy was far from the only one who was way ahead of the game. In 1956, Surgeon-Captain TL Cleave, MRCP, formerly Director of Medical Research of the Institute of Naval Medicine in the UK, went as far as to say that 'the saccharine disease' was the 'master disease'. He explained that this master disease incorporated diabetes, coronary disease, varicose veins, *E coli* infections, obesity, constipation, haemorrhoids, appendicitis – and that's just to start with.

Dr Cleave and his associates noted:

There is one common factor in all traditional healthy diets: the absence of sugar and all simple carbohydrates.

Simple carbohydrates – that's refined sugar and flour!

Even the man who discovered insulin, Dr Frederick Banting, tried to tell the world in 1929 that his discovery was *not* a cure at all, and that the only way to prevent diabetes was to cut down on 'dangerous' sugar bingeing:

In the US the incidence of diabetes has increased proportionately with the per capita consumption of sugar.

Unfortunately, his advice fell on deaf ears, and most people, even to this day, are blind to the truth about sugar. Sadly this isn't just a figure of speech; many people have literally been blinded by sugar. Sugar is seen as something which might make you fat and rot your teeth, but few know its full harmful potential. You might think of diabetes as a slightly unfortunate condition where people suffer the inconvenience of either having to inject insulin a few times a day (type 1) or to control their diet a bit. What may come as a bit of an eye-opener is that many people lose their sight and their limbs as a direct result of diabetes, a disease which nine times out of ten is *directly* caused by the over-consumption of refined sugars and carbohydrates.

I watched an extremely graphic programme about sugar which showed how one woman became blind in her early 30s simply because of her addiction to refined sugar-laced 'foods'. It must be extremely hard to swallow if you get cancer because you smoke, but to go blind because of a 'sweet tooth' must be devastating. At least these days, smokers have some degree of warning to the possible dangers; all the sugar eater/addict knows is that eating too much *may* contribute to weight gain – they are none the wiser to the dangers exposed by Dr Cleave and Dr Banting. Even today there are still no provisions in place to put warnings on labels of refined carbohydrates.

The problem is that people see refined sugars and carbohydrates, unlike cigarettes, as food, not as nutrition-less, highly additive, disease-causing rubbish. If there's one thing I want to hammer home in this book it is that

Refined sugars and carbohydrates are *not* food!

They have been stripped of their nutritional content and supply only empty calories, which in turn soon make us feel the same – empty. You cannot expect to feel fulfilled when you are eating and drinking empty 'foods'.

Your Insulin Bank Account

Every time you eat refined carbohydrates, your body goes into emergency mode. Because all the vitamins, minerals and fibre have been stripped out, the sugars have no 'buffer' and enter the bloodstream too rapidly. This causes a major imbalance in the fine workings of the system, and the body needs to act *fast* in order to survive. If sugar levels rise too high and stay there, you die – that's how important it is for the body to do whatever it can to fix the immediate danger. It does this by producing insulin in the pancreas, which rushes through the bloodstream and 'burns' off the excess sugar (or energy).

So what's the problem?

First, and I believe most important, you are born with only so much insulin in your insulin bank account. If you keep making withdrawals the organ can easily 'burn out' and stop producing sufficient amounts of insulin for the job in hand. When this happens you have diabetes and your pancreas will simply never be the same again.

Second, insulin is known as the 'FAT-PRODUCING' hormone. The excess energy which was burnt off in the bloodstream by the insulin has to go somewhere. The first places are the liver and muscles for short-term energy use, but once those stores are full it transports the excess directly into FAT CELLS.

Clearly, if you exercise you will burn off the excess calories, and fat won't be a problem for you. It also won't be a problem if you don't eat that much; even if it is refined carbs. However, even if you do burn it off and you are slim, your pancreas and other vital organs are still getting a beating. You are still susceptible to what Dr Cleave described as the 'saccharine disease', a disease that encompasses just about every degenerative disease you can think of.

But even before diabetes sets in, your pancreas can easily begin to malfunction. For many, this is a major cause of their overeating and weight gain. The problem with a malfunctioning pancreas is that it overproduces insulin, causing far too much of the fat-producing hormone to pour into the bloodstream at once. When this happens, you have elevated levels of insulin in your bloodstream causing you to feel empty, dissatisfied and hungry. This in turn can easily cause someone to overeat in a desperate attempt to feel full.

This is why so many people, the minute they start to eat, feel hungrier than before they took the first bite. How many times have you heard people say, 'Oh, I didn't realize I was that hungry'? The problem is they weren't *that* hungry until a surge of insulin was released into the bloodstream.

Double Whammy

The pancreas can malfunction to such an extent that the bloodstream has *permanently* elevated levels of insulin. This means you have a constant degree of dissatisfaction and a feeling of emptiness. It also causes another problem:

When you have elevated levels of insulin in your bloodstream it not only promotes fat storage but also prevents *already-stored* fat from being broken down.

This means that a person who is already overweight and has a malfunctioning pancreas wouldn't need to 'pig out' to get bigger or to fail to lose weight. In these cases, cutting down a *little* on refined carbohydrates often fails to help on the fat front. What's needed is a total refined-sugar cleanse.

The Sugar Illusion

The sudden rises in sugar levels are, like any drug reaction, soon followed by a low – in this case a sugar low. And when you have a sugar low, no amount of tuna salad is going to cut the mustard – your brain and body demands more SUGAR! Unless sugar eaters get their next fix, they're not happy bunnies; and when they do have their fix the 'addictive' side comes into play. Because their sugar levels are lifted when they consume more sugar (or refined carbohydrates), they *instantly* feel much better than they did a moment earlier. This gives the false impression that it's more 'fun' to eat junk than it is to eat veggies, fruit, fish and salad.

But what all sugar heads must understand is that the instant 'pleasure' only manifests itself because of the low; without the low there would be no contrast. This is the equivalent of picking up heavy shopping and holding it for a while for the sole purpose of getting the pleasure of putting it down, or watching *EastEnders* in order to feel intelligent! The degree of pleasure the sugar addict feels is an illusion, and it takes an incredibly open-minded person to see it. But because the sugar illusion is so subtle and because, until pointed out, most people cannot see it, those who do not indulge are seen as boring no-hopers.

Actress Halle Berry has perhaps one of the healthiest eating and health regimes there are, yet time and again she is slagged off for being boring *purely* because of what she chooses to eat and drink. One of the supplements in *OK!* magazine gave the following quote from Halle: 'I eat healthily and I don't eat fried foods. I only get sugar through fruit and veg', after which they printed their own comment: 'Zzz … boring!' But how the flipping blazes is she being boring just because she doesn't eat refined sugar? It's this type of nonsensical comment which helps fuel the false belief that eating refined sugar is in some way exciting and fun; along with clever advertising telling us 'It's pleasure we can't measure' or certain foods can 'take us to paradise' or we can 'thank Crunchie it's Friday'. I don't know about you, but whenever I'm feeling pissed off about something I can eat all the sugary foods in the world and I still feel pissed off. The only difference is that I now also feel guilty, fat and anxious.

All other creatures on the planet get their sugars _only_ from the natural foods they eat. Refined sugar just doesn't exist in the wild.

And coincidentally, neither does eating as a response to emotion, diabetes, overweight, or mental addiction! After only a few days of eating and drinking the right foods and getting a good blast of daily oxygen on the 14-day programme, the sugar rollercoaster you may have been on for years will come to an end. You don't need to remove all carbohydrates from your diet, but if you really want to take your health to the next level, this member of the Seven Deadly Dietary Sins must be drastically cut down or removed completely.

I realize that removing refined sugars from your diet _completely_ may prove more than tricky, especially as sugar is hidden in almost everything, but as you will be eating mainly live foods, good _wholegrain_ carbohydrates and lean proteins, it will be much easier than you think. And if you are free of diet mentality, then it's frighteningly easy.

2. Refined Fats

As you will read in the Six Essential Dietary Needs, fat is an absolute necessity for optimum health (page 145). But it's critical that it's the right kind of fat – and the word critical really isn't out of place when talking about the wrong fats!

We have known for some time that the wrong kinds of fats can be bad for us, but many think the worst culprit is saturated fat, found mainly in animal products. However, saturated fat is almost like a breath of fresh air compared with the ugliest fat of them all:

HYDROGENATED VEGETABLE FAT

Please remember the above and embed it into your mind so that a) you never forget it and b) you never knowingly eat anything which contains it. While you're there, also remember these words: 'deodorized', 'winterized', 'bleached', 'refined', 'trans fats' and 'trans fatty acids' – all of which mean pretty much the same thing. Many vegetarians and vegans are under the terrible misapprehension that, not eating animal fat, they are hunky-dory on the cholesterol front. Nothing could be further from the truth.

When you heat vegetable oils and fats to high temperatures you turn something which was originally classed as 'healthy' into a substance that can only be described as *extremely* dangerous. In order to produce fats and oils which do not turn rancid, manufacturers subject them to enormous heat – anything up to 1000°F. Hydrogen is bubbled through the oil and forced under pressure into the boiling fat molecules. When fats and oils have been heat-treated to this degree, virtually all the naturally occurring nutrients are lost, including the *essential* fatty acids. Not only are the good fats more or less destroyed by exposing fats and oils to these sorts of high temperatures, but the whole molecular structure has changed to such a degree that the fats and oils become harmful. Hydrogenated oil or 'trans fat' can create a build-up of LDL (low-density lipoprotein) cholesterol (the bad one). LDL molecules squeeze beneath the blood-vessel linings and narrow the passageways with a layer of 'plaque'. This has been found to be a *major* cause of **heart disease** and **cancer**.

This kind of fat is so harmful that US government experts declared *'there is no safe level of consumption'*, and are strongly considering putting warning labels on foods containing trans fats. Clearly, there is a safe level of consumption, otherwise people would keel over after one slice of cake, but the cumulative effect is perhaps what they meant.

Understanding is Child's Play

To get a better picture of what's happening when you eat foods containing hydrogenated fats and oils, think of those children's learning toys where you have a board from which different shapes have been cut out. Now imagine someone giving you a completely different set of shapes and asking you to try and fit each one in the holes provided. This is precisely what you are asking your body to do when you eat trans-fatty acids. Actually, it's even worse as the wrong shapes often get wedged into the wrong holes, preventing the right shapes from ever getting to where they belong. This means that even if you eat good fats and oils you could still be suffering from an essential fatty-acid deficiency if your system is full of trans fats.

Not Worth a Sausage

Trans fats are found in many foods, from baked goods to mass-market chocolate. But did you know they are also in many 'health' foods. There's nothing wrong with becoming vegetarian, but very few vegetarians actually eat many vegetables! Their diet often consists mainly of refined breads, pastries, pasta, cakes, or foods that look or taste like meat. Over the past 20 years there has been an explosion of 'vegetarian' sausages, burgers, Kievs and roasts. If people are eating these instead of meat for animal-rights issues then fair play, but if they have switched for health reasons then their thinking is flawed.

If you look at the label of your average 'meat-free' packet you will usually see the words 'hydrogenated vegetable oil'. You will also see the same thing written on many 'vegetarian-friendly' snacks such as flapjacks and cakes. These fats and oils are much *more* harmful to your health than saturated fat. In fact, there's not that much evidence to show that saturated fat is anywhere near as bad as we have been taught (see below).

This doesn't mean for a second that 'real' sausages or burgers are good. In fact, I call run-of-the-mill sausages and burgers 'mystery food', as it's a complete mystery what's in them! I'm also not suggesting that you should go back to eating meat if you are a vegetarian; I'm just pointing out that many vegetarian ready-made foods are full of trans fats and are therefore more detrimental to your health than the fats found in meat.

Saturated with Lies

Saturated fat – just the words are usually enough to squeeze any artery into submission, but the reason we are scared of saturated fat is purely down to what we've heard. The truth, however, is that saturated fat, cholesterol and heart disease may not be as linked as we think. Over half the calories in mother's milk, for example, are in the form of fat, much of it saturated fat. Mother's milk also has a higher proportion of cholesterol than almost any other food. Most people don't realize that both cholesterol and saturated fat are essential for growth in babies, especially for the development of the brain. Much of the fat found in fresh coconuts is saturated, but there's no way that coconuts, or the milk they contain, are harmful to the human body. It's not so much saturated fat that's the problem: it's the *refined* fats we replace them with in the name of 'health'.

Numerous studies over the years have shown clearly that saturated fat is not the bad fat it is purported to be. One such study compared Jews living in Yemen, who got their fats purely from animal-origin diets, with Yemenite Jews living in Israel, whose dietary fats came from margarine and vegetable oils. The first group revealed little heart disease or diabetes, but the second group had high levels of both. A more important part of the study, though, was that the Yemenite Jews also consumed no sugar, whereas those in Israel ate over a quarter of their carbohydrate intake as sugar.

The Japanese have the longest lifespan of any nationality. Most people put this down to their low-fat diet, but although the Japanese eat very few dairy fats, they do eat quite a lot of saturated fat. Most dishes have animal fats in the form of eggs, pork, chicken, beef, fish and shellfish. In fact, they probably eat more seafood than any other nation, all of which contains cholesterol. Once again, they do not eat a lot of trans fats, vegetable oil, white flour and refined sugar. I'm not saying that animal fats are good or in any way better than those found in plant foods – because they're not. I'm just pointing out that when it comes to the Seven Deadly Dietary Sins, it's REFINED FATS and not so much saturated fats that get top billing.

As always, though, be guided by common sense and your gut instinct. When you see egg and bacon swimming around in fat in a frying pan, common sense should tell you that it will do you much more harm than a piece of lean grilled chicken. In fact, there's no evidence to show that a lean piece of grilled chicken will do any harm to a well-functioning digestive system. Heating and frying oils changes the molecule structure and turns what are sometimes good fats into incredibly dangerous ones. If you have a choice between 'real' sausages and vegetarian sausages, have an avocado!

3. Alcohol

Not a food, true, but alcohol is certainly a major part of many people's diets – especially in the UK and Ireland. And when you think how many people there are who say they *only* drink Guinness for the iron and wine for the antioxidants, plus many doctors and newspaper reports claiming alcohol is 'good' for you, I simply couldn't leave it out.

Now alcohol may or may not be a problem for you. One way to know for certain is if the thought of *never* drinking it again fills you with fear and makes you panic about how you would enjoy yourself or handle stress. If it does then it's time you faced up to a fact you may not like – you're hooked!

The following section may not convince you to stop drinking, but as you are going to be doing without alcohol during the 14-day Turbo-charge Your Life programme, the facts below may help to make it easier for you.

Alcohol is *Not* Good for You!

Let me make something very clear – alcohol is not good for you; and yes, that even includes red wine! Of all the things that have ever been written about alcohol, the one about its health benefits has got to take the biscuit. Remember that 'experts' told us smoking was good for us at one point too, so please be open-minded to the possibility that they could have been wrong.

First, alcohol is a poison. It is more toxic to the human body than heroin. Let me repeat that in case it passed you by:

ALCOHOL IS MORE TOXIC THAN HEROIN

Alcohol also increases blood pressure, acts as a depressant and destroys brain cells. When you drink alcohol you literally pound the brain; it's like going into a boxing ring every weekend (or, for some, every night!) and deliberately hitting yourself on the head over and over again. A nurse friend of mine informed me that she was once present at something called a 'Commando operation'. The operation was on a man who had a tumour on the side of his face. It had spread so much that they had to remove virtually the side of his face plus part of his head. This exposed his brain during the operation. The surgeon said that the man was obviously a heavy drinker. My friend asked how he knew. He asked her to look at the size of the brain; it was a lot smaller than it was meant to be. This, he informed her, was a direct result of the patient's drinking. In plain English:

ALCOHOL SHRINKS THE BRAIN!

Alcohol Came First – Kebabs Second!

On top of all that, alcohol is a major contributor to weight-gain. So much so that many people lose tremendous amounts of weight just by eliminating alcohol alone. But I'm not concerned just with the weight-gain caused by the alcohol itself; it's all the stuff we eat because of alcohol that helps to cause disease and pile on the pounds. Alcohol causes dehydration and low blood sugar, creating cravings for stodgy fats and refined carbohydrates. This is why you see kebab shops and chippies packed with people at 11pm on Friday and Saturday nights and why people tuck into a fry-up the next morning.

You Don't Drink! But How Do You Live?

Alcohol is a subject all in itself and there is no way I can even begin to explain the full nature of this beast and the degree of 'hook' it has over our nation, but one thing I would suggest is that during the 14-day programme you make a point of going out to have a non-drink so that you can see first-hand how this liquid drug has a nation in its clutches. It is only when you are not drinking that you can see the full impact of alcohol.

I was helping to run what could be described as a Turbo-Charge Your Life event in Tenerife along with some fellow 'coaches' who happen not to drink. Whilst we were there we decided to go out and hit the town a few times. To those who have been to resorts like Las Americas in Tenerife you will know that as you walk around there are young girls and boys trying to lure you into their particular bar in order to get some commission on the drinks. As we wandered around we were stopped almost every minute by someone asking us if we wanted a 'two for one' deal on certain alcoholic drinks. When we said thanks but we don't drink some of the answers came even as a shock to me. One girl said, with a look of shock on her face as she stared at our water bottles, 'But how on earth do you live?' – and she meant it! Another girl was left virtually speechless, saying after a long pause, 'well … I … really don't know what to say to that. I have been working here all summer and I've never heard a group of people say they don't drink.'

If you think this happened only because it was in a holiday resort I can assure you the same thing happens whenever you nip out.

Alcohol is the only drug on the planet that you have to justify *not* taking.

You will find this over the next 14 days when you go out, and I urge you to treat it like a game. Even if you have no intention of stopping drinking for ever, just say to everyone that you no longer drink and watch the reaction. This just proves how much of a hold it has over people. If I decided to stop eating apples and my friends didn't, I doubt if I would get a load of abuse, but with alcohol – my God! The best way to floor people is to say, '*I'm sorry I don't drink when I'm sober*' – that's usually enough to fry their brain for a second.

If you do go out and enjoy your non-drink nights and don't moan about not having alcohol (as people do when they're 'on the wagon'), you may well find that you don't want to go back after the 14 days – sobriety really can be that addictive.

If you feel as though you have a degree of alcohol problem which cannot be dealt with the tools in this book, then please may I strongly suggest you get hold of *Stop Drinking 4 Life … Easily* (go to www.juicemaster.com and click on shopping).

4. Artificial Sweeteners

Many people are still under the terrible misapprehension that artificial sweeteners are in some way better than sugar. However, not only are many sweeteners just as bad as the real thing, but some research shows they are often even worse – and if you're taking them to help with weight loss you could well be on a hiding to nothing.

Sweet Fat Lies

Dr Ralph Walton, Professor of the Department of Psychiatry at Northeast Ohio University's College of Medicine, believes the calorie-saving advantage of artificial sweeteners is totally thwarted because it makes people prone to binge eating. He states:

If you feed a laboratory animal aspartame, you wind up with an obese animal.

Aspartame, more commonly known as NutraSweet, is one of the most widely used sweeteners. He continues by giving some pretty clear advice on the subject:

If you are trying to lose weight, you should stay away from aspartame.

Betty Martin, a leading US food and safety campaigner, is equally scathing:

We see literally thousands of cases of people who have been taking aspartame for a long time, and they are always overweight. Aspartame actually makes you crave carbohydrates so you **gain** weight.

It's a No-brainer

Weight gain, however, seems like a picnic compared with some of the other symptoms which have been linked to artificial sweeteners. Aspartame has been associated with 92 different symptoms including headaches, poor vision, depression, panic attacks, irregular heart rhythms, behavioural problems, seizures and, most worrying of all, brain tumours! This isn't just hearsay from a few nuts on the internet either. One senior FDA (Food and Drug Administration) toxicologist said:

At least one test has established beyond reasonable doubt that aspartame is capable of producing brain tumours in animals.

The Surgeon General, head of public health in the US, said he believes aspartame usage to be a major contributing factor to the mental disorders suffered by 22 million Americans.

Clearly, the amount of artificial sweetener contained in one can of diet fizzy drink isn't enough to cause the 92 symptoms linked to some artificial sweeteners, but then one cigarette isn't enough to cause cancer or emphysema. That doesn't mean that the *cumulative* effect won't cause these problems. And, like cigarettes, it appears there is a degree of addiction associated with artificial sweeteners. So how do you know if something contains artificial sweetener? First point of call is to check the label, but the words 'SUGAR FREE' are a more obvious sign. Ninety-nine times out of a hundred, 'sugar free' means 'contains artificial sweeteners'.

Such is the financial lure of the 'sugar-free' market, new artificial sweeteners are making their way into food and drinks all the time. Artificial sweeteners can now be found in almost everything: drinks, foods, gums, vitamin tablets and even baby foods! However, no matter what the sweetener, or how safe the claim, you can bet your bottom dollar that as the years go on it will come out that they aren't as safe as we once thought.

On the 14-day programme, the idea is not to switch to artificial sweeteners from sugar, but to retrain your taste buds to love foods and drinks without sweeteners or sugar.

5. Caffeine

Caffeine is found in tea and coffee, and 90 per cent of us drink one or the other or both, often to excess. However, after I give you some home truths on the caffeine front I can guarantee you will choose at least to cut down considerably on the two most-used 'drink drugs'.

The Age-old Story

Caffeine is extremely toxic to the human body. So much so that when it enters the bloodstream, the body sees it as a foreign invader and goes into emergency mode, firing off the adrenal glands. Every time the adrenal glands are triggered into action, it speeds up the ageing process. The adrenal glands were designed to be fired in 'emergency' situations – like being attacked by a wild animal; it's the 'fight or flight' mechanism. The body was designed to deal thousands of true 'emergency' moments; what Nature didn't expect, however, was that we would drink a substance several times a day that would have the same impact on our systems as being attacked by a rhino!

Every time you drink a cup of coffee or tea (or soft drinks like Red Bull and Coke) you jolt your nervous system and dehydrate your body. This creates an almost constant state of stress – your kidneys and liver take a battering, you overwork your adrenal glands and you rob your brain and body of water.

Are You Taking the Pee?

Caffeine is a strong diuretic – meaning it makes you pee. The biggest problem with this is that if you keep dehydrating your body, the kidneys will conserve water by making less urine. As a result, the urine becomes highly concentrated, which leads to crystals separating out. These crystals can eventually build up and produce KIDNEY STONES.

For those who have never had the complete displeasure of suffering from kidney stones, from what I have been told by several people, it's something you really do want to pass on.

Another Weighty Problem

Weight loss is most people's number-one concern when changing their eating and drinking habits. Caffeine is usually the last thing to leave the diet because people believe it has no effect on the weight front. However, like artificial sweeteners, caffeine can stimulate cravings for sugar – the very thing that causes the majority of weight gain. It's worth knowing that:

When caffeine hits the central nervous system it *lowers* blood sugar, which *increases* the brain's demand for more *sugar*.

On top of this, ever since the famous 'Central Perk' in *Friends*, we have 'hip 'n' trendy' coffee bars popping up all over the place selling, not coffee as we know it, but more of a warm, creamy coffee milkshake. Did you know there are now twice as many Starbucks on the Island of Manhattan as there are McDonald's? To put this in real perspective you need to understand that there are more Ronald establishments in New York City *per capita* than anywhere else in the US – no wonder they call it Star*bucks*!

I stopped drinking coffee many years ago and as my taste buds have changed so much, the taste of 'real' coffee is something I now hate. However, I made the error of trying a Starbucks vanilla latte one cold, damp, dark evening after a friend told me I couldn't judge places like Starbucks until I had tried one myself. I kept saying I wouldn't like it as I hate coffee now, but I soon discovered that what I had ordered was perhaps a world away from how 'real' coffee tastes. It was sweet, creamy and warm – a combination that really did (and I hate to admit this) taste good. So I do know that for many people reading this doing without your daily 'hip 'n' trendy' may be something you aren't looking forward to.

However, as I will keep mentioning throughout the book, the programme is only for 14 days and you can then make a lifetime judgement about coffee *after* that time. Many people, even those classed as 'heavy user' in the 'hip 'n' trendy' coffee world, find that after the Turbo-charge programme (and often just after the first 3–4 days into it) their desire for the dark stuff has dropped dramatically. Many people never touch the stuff again after the programme (and don't miss it) and some find they have the odd one here and there but their 'daily' need has vanished.

However, what may help is a word from Dr David Kerr, of the Royal Bournemouth Hospital, summing up the harmful effects of caffeine:

Within half an hour of drinking one or two cups, the flow of blood to the brain is reduced by 10–20 per cent. Combine that with low blood sugar and you can soon start to have palpitations, feelings of anxiety or blurred vision.

Easy to Kick It

One of the reasons why people find it much, much easier after the first few days without caffeine is not only because they are adjusting mentally, but because it only takes 48 to 72 hours for caffeine to leave the system. In reality almost all of the addictive qualities are psychological, meaning once your brain is happy to kick the substance into touch, you will hardly notice any physical discomfort. The average caffeine drinker will probably not be aware of any withdrawal symptoms, as long as they drink plenty of water and freshly extracted juices, and eat plenty of water-rich foods. The most they can expect is a slight headache and perhaps some feelings of anxiety.

6. Salt

If you are thirsty and stranded on a dingy in the middle of the ocean, one thing you should never do is drink the water surrounding you. Why? Because the salt content will dehydrate you so much that you will die more quickly! Salt, as we know it, is not only unnecessary but also detrimental to your health. According to studies, if food manufacturers cut the salt they used by half, 100,000 lives a year could be saved in the UK.

White refined table salt contains highly toxic sodium. When refined salt enters the body the kidneys have to work their socks off to get rid of it. This means lots more blood is pumped through the kidneys, and the end result is hypertension (high blood pressure). High Blood Pressure = Heart Disease and Strokes. The massive increase in refined salt in everyday foods is having alarming effects. Children as young as four are showing signs of changes in their veins and arteries similar to those found in the early stages of hypertension. It may be highly illegal to add nicotine to anything a child may come into contact with, but something like refined salt seems fair game.

I can only assume that the people who tell us we need this kind of salt in order to survive must have some sort of vested interest in doing so, or of course they have left their common sense behind. Natural sodium we need – the small amounts Nature provides in nearly all fruits, vegetables, nuts and fish – but refined salt we don't need at all. As much as 75 per cent of dietary salt comes from processed foods. The biggest contributors are bread, breakfast cereals, biscuits, cakes, rice, flour and pasta. Every time you eat a sandwich, a pasty, a flapjack, a bun, a baguette or a muffin you are eating salt.

Over **220,000 TONS OF SALT** are added to *all sorts* of processed food *every year* in the **UK ALONE.**

Sir John Krebs, chairman of the FSA (Food Standards Agency), said:

High blood pressure really is the silent killer. The human cost in terms of illness and death and the costs to the NHS are very high ... Cutting down on salt can significantly reduce your risk of developing high blood pressure.

Those with high blood pressure are three times more likely to develop heart disease and stroke, and twice as likely to die from these diseases. So if salt is so bad, why do food manufacturers insist on adding tons of the stuff to their food? First, it's a great preservative – the Egyptians even used it for preserving dead bodies! Second, it causes dehydration, which many food companies love as they also have interests in the soft-drinks market. And third, it's a cheap and addictive ingredient.

7. Dairy Products

Many of you may be surprised to see dairy in this section. Due to the incredible amount of brainwashing about how 'good' dairy apparently is, you may well have expected to find dairy products in The Six Essential Dietary Needs. In order to get a clear grasp of why dairy is in this section, you need to put aside everything you have been taught and just begin to use your common sense.

Open Your Mind

If doctors, dieticians, parents, teachers and the government all say dairy is not only good but an essential part of our diet, then who are we mere mortals to question it? But if you do question it, you will discover that making dairy an entire 'essential group' on its own was about the craziest ever piece of nutritional advice. If there are any qualified dieticians or closed-minded nutritionists out there who still hold the view that dairy is simply the best source of calcium and protein for the body, please do yourself a favour and read this with an open mind.

Cows Don't Drink Milk – So Why Do We?

We are the only mammals on the planet that still drink milk after weaning age. If you think about it, even a cow doesn't drink milk – calves do, but not cows. That's because it's extremely unnatural for any mammal to drink milk of any kind after they have been weaned, and it's even more unnatural to drink the milk from an entirely different species. Cow's milk, was specifically designed for a mammal with *four* stomachs – we have *one*.

But What About My Calcium?

What about it? If you think it through, we are the only mammals with calcium deficiencies such as brittle-bone disease (osteoporosis) and tooth-loss. If you are thinking that cats and dogs also suffer from calcium-deficiency diseases, please bear in mind who controls what they eat. I'm talking here about wild mammals; mammals that *never* eat processed food and eat only food designed for them by Nature – which, funnily enough, doesn't include dairy products.

Doesn't it strike you as slightly odd? If milk and dairy are as good for our bones as we have been conditioned to believe, then why has the incidence of osteoporosis *increased* dramatically over the past 50 years? Also, why has this happened at exactly the same time as we are consuming more dairy products than ever before? I don't think you need a degree in common sense to deduce that what we were told may have been just a little way from the truth. The fact is, dairy products are *not* vital for good bone health. As Dr Tierry Burn says:

The Chinese consume no cow's milk or dairy products, yet they have among the lowest rates of osteoporosis in the world.

Another fact that seems to have flown by dairy fans is that *all* fruit and veg contain 'usable' calcium, with dark-green leafy veg such as broccoli, spinach and kale being particularly rich sources. The humble onion is your best bet against weak bones. A study from the University of Bern in Switzerland found that just one gram of onion a day is enough to strengthen your skeleton.

Casein Versus Calcium

It's true that milk contains calcium, but then so do oyster shells. Just because something contains a substance we know to be good doesn't necessarily mean it's in the best form for a human. After all, there are plenty of minerals in food which can also be found in many rock faces, but I seriously doubt that Nature intended us to get our magnesium or zinc from this source. Equally, just because protein and calcium can be found in cow's milk, they may not be in a form conducive to human digestion.

As well as calcium, milk contains a protein called casein. The casein and calcium are chemically bound together. In order for the protein to be used efficiently and the calcium to be utilized properly, the body requires certain digestive enzymes to split them up. These enzymes are called rennin and lactase. Here's the rub – most humans stop producing these enzymes after the age of three or four. Because of this, the human body would have a degree of difficulty dealing with even *human* milk after weaning age, but when you start drinking cow's milk the body really can be in trouble.

Cow's milk contains over 300 times more casein than human milk. Just to let you in on why this is not a good thing: casein is used as a base in one of the strongest glues.

It sticks to the walls of the stomach and the lining of the intestines. How many times have you heard people say, 'I'm going to have a few beers tonight, but before I do I'm going to line my stomach with milk'? That is exactly what's happening – your stomach and intestines are being covered with a glue-like substance. This can cause all kinds of problems, from food not being absorbed properly, creating an acidic reaction in the body, to the common milk and dairy symptom of mucus build-up.

More and more people are being diagnosed with an intolerance to milk and dairy products. It has been proved to be a major contributing factor in diseases like asthma, hay fever and eczema. This shouldn't come as any great surprise as cow's milk is a 'foreign invader' to an adult human digestive system, and in many cases there will be some kind of inflammatory response to deal with the problem.

Now unlike nicotine, alcohol, trans fats, salt and refined sugars, milk is not going kill you, even taking into account the cumulative effect.

However, it does play a part in clogging the system and lowering immunity, which then contributes to all kinds of diseases. However, unlike other members of The Seven Dietary Sins, dairy products aren't necessarily addictive. This means the occasional dip into the dairy pot is fine.

So is my best bet to become vegan?

There's really no need to go vegan for health reasons unless you have a mucus-forming problem (asthma, hay fever, bronchitis or eczema). So if you want some butter on your jacket potato – don't lose sleep! The body will get *some* goodness from dairy.

Alive and Kicking

One exception on the dairy front is 'live' yoghurts. Live yoghurts have 'friendly bacteria' which break down the lactose (milk sugar) and the casein (protein). This means the two main dietary concerns about dairy are not a problem. Live yogurts are also of great benefit for those with fungal problems such as *Candida albicans*, thrush and athlete's foot. When buying live yogurts, always make sure they are natural and sweeten with fruit such as berries.

Common 'Foods' and 'Drinks' to Avoid from the Seven Deadly Dietary Sins

All fried food (except stir-fried)

All traditional fast-food 'joints'

All white-flour carbohydrates

Anything with 'simple' refined sugars, refined fats or refined salts

Anything with hydrogenated vegetable oil or trans fats

Baked goods

Beer and lager

Biscuits

Blue cheese

Cakes

Canned foods (most are full of sugar and salt)

Carton juices

Chips

Chocolate (except Fair Trade 85% cocoa)

Coffee and tea

Cow's milk

Crisps

Fizzy sodas (Coke, Sprite, etc.)

Hot chocolate (sorry!)

Ice cream

Muffins

Pork – very bad one!

Preserves, jams, marmalade, etc.

Ready meals – most are loaded with refined salts, fats and sugars
  (check the label!)

Red meat

Roasted and salted nuts

Sweets (candy)

Table salt

Wheat-based bread and pasta

Yellow cheese

Yoghurts (other than 'live', organic, free from sugar and sweeteners
  – the best I've found is the Rachel's Organic Range)

Nicotine

Technically not a food or a drink, but I've included nicotine, or smoking if you will, in the Seven Deadly Dietary Sins because it is something people put into their mouths and it is something people, mainly teenage girls, believe acts as an aid to keeping slim. Because of this I felt it should go in with the 'real' Seven Deadly Dietary Sins. As you will see, if we count nicotine, there are actually eight sins here, but nicotine really stands alone in the world and so technically is not part of the main seven.

Smoking clearly isn't good for you; I think you'd have had to have had your head in the sand for the past 20 years not to know this. Not only is smoking just 'not good for you', but the average cigarette contains over 4000 chemicals, many of which are a direct cause of cancer.

However, even armed with this fact, I know so many smokers who are not just a little funny about their food, but *insist* on 'organic' foods and drinks. These are some people who will be extremely careful not to put too many pesticides, fungicides, sugar or 'junk' into their bodies, yet inhaling 4000 chemicals every half an hour doesn't seem to bother them.

I'm actually being a tad facetious as being a former two- to three-packet-a-day smoker myself, I'm more than aware of this lifestyle contradiction. I was even teaching aerobics at the same as smoking 40–60 cigarettes a day! This doesn't mean for a millisecond that good quality nutrition means nothing if you smoke; the reality is it means even more. So even if you have no intention of stopping smoking at this time, you will still gain tremendous mental and physical benefits on the Turbo-charge Your Life programme.

The truth is that when it comes to addiction all reason goes out of the window. Nicotine, whether it's contained in a cigarette, cigar or pipe, is one of, if not the most, addictive drug on the planet and like all drugs it causes a mental tug-of-war in the addict. One side of the brain can easily see it for the expensive, filthy, disease-causing nightmare that it is and would love more than anything to stop doing it, whereas the irrational 'drug-addicted' side simply cannot imagine life without the drug and so wants to continue. This causes a constant mental battle and is the reason why smokers spend most of their lives either smoking wishing they weren't doing it or not smoking wishing that they could do it! It also causes the lifestyle contradiction for many of insisting on buying organic foods but smoking at the same time.

Smokers Are Not Stupid!

Despite what it may look like to non-smokers, smokers are not stupid. All smokers are more than fully aware of exactly how much they cost and what harm they can do to their short- and long-term health. In other words, all smokers know exactly why they shouldn't smoke. However, what they don't know is why they do smoke. On the surface, smokers will think they know why they smoke and will come up with all kinds of what they believe to be legitimate reasons, such as: it helps me to relax; it aids concentration; it's enjoyable; it's a reward; it relieves boredom. However, what they don't realize is that the only reason why they smoke is to try to relieve the empty, insecure feeling caused, ironically, by the last cigarette they smoked!

As soon as a smoker finishes a cigarette, nicotine starts to leave the body immediately. Nicotine levels drop to about half within one to two hours. When this happens it causes an empty, insecure feeling in the bloodstream, a feeling which is immediately relieved by lighting up another cigarette. The smoker is then tricked into believing the cigarette helps to relieve some kind of genuine life-related feeling, when all it's doing is getting rid of the feeling the last cigarette caused. In truth even that's not correct as when you smoke a cigarette all you are doing is partially relieving the feeling as the body has built up an immunity and tolerance to the drug over the years. The pleasure the smoker thinks they would miss if they stopped is not real and is akin to the pleasure you get when putting down some heavy shopping. Sure it's heaven, but who in their right mind would ever pick up some heavy bags, walk around in them all day simply to get the pleasure of putting them down again?

The problem is, because the smoker is being so cleverly deluded by the drug itself, they cannot see what is actually happening, which is why smoking contradicts so many other aspects of their lives. I know this first hand as I was pretty much in control of most things in my life, yet I couldn't get to grips with a silly paper tube stuffed with all sorts of chemicals.

Stopping Smoking Can Be Very Easy!

Despite what you may have heard, it only actually takes 3 days for all of the nicotine to leave the body – regardless of how many someone smokes or how long they've been smoking. And the irritability people suffer when they stop is NOT, as many people – including doctors – believe, primarily caused by nicotine withdrawal itself but more by a mental insecurity of being without what they believe is their crutch.

The only way to quit is when you put out your final cigarette you need to understand at that moment you are not in the process of stopping – you've already stopped. This is the biggest mistake people make after they stop: they wait to see how long it will take to believe they are free. The problem is this could take for ever as it's only when they say 'Thank God I'm Free' that they are truly free – so why don't they just say it right from the start?

As long as they don't moan about not having a cigarette, don't envy other smokers and see stopping as an amazing and liberating thing, they will find the physical withdrawal almost imperceptible.

The main reason why smokers find it difficult to stop is because they still mope around for cigarettes after they stop. These are the same cigarettes don't forget that they wanted to get rid of: the same cigarettes which were enslaving them, killing them, making them look like a social lepers, causing them to age fast, not to mention costing them a fortune. This means they stop smoking – which was meant to be a good and liberating thing – but then cause themselves a problem by moping around for the very things which they hope they will no longer have. Think about it – that really is a few butts short of a full ashtray isn't it? To mope around, to get yourself angry and upset because you no longer have the very thing you wanted to get rid of.

I realize that a simple page on nicotine will rarely help someone to stop smoking, but then on the other hand, why shouldn't it? If you use the other information contained in this book, the job could be done right now. The only thing that is preventing a smoker from putting out their final cigarette and jumping for joy that they are free from the blooming nasty things is them. If they wanted to, I mean really wanted to, they could make the decision to quit right now. They could set a date, get mentally prepared, put out their final cigarette on that day and finally end the one-way life-draining relationship. After all, even if someone finds it hard, how hard is it compared with what Lance Armstrong, Michael Watson or Christopher Reeve were willing to go through in order to achieve what they wanted? At this stage I feel it necessary to remind you of a Lance Armstrong quote: 'Pain is temporary; quitting lasts a lifetime.' In this case the quote is very apt as quitting, when it comes to smoking, is something you actually want to last a lifetime. What you don't want is the lifelong pain of quitting trying to stop. Even if you do feel a degree of what you perceive as mental 'pain' for a few days, remember it's only temporary – quitting lasts a lifetime.

If you need further assistance on this or think 'one thing at a time Jason, come on!', then either get hold of the 'Stop Smoking in 2 Hours' double-CD programme, attend a Stop Smoking session with myself or one of my trainers, or get hold of *Stop Smoking 4 Life … EASILY!* (See website www.juice-master.com) or come to the clinic for a session – call 0845 1 30 28 29.

CIGARETTES CONTAIN OVER 4000 CHEMICALS: MORE THAN 40 OF THEM ARE KNOWN TO CAUSE CANCER

Tobacco firms have admitted putting 600 secret ingredients and additives in cigarettes the Health Secretary disclosed yesterday … The ingredients include sucrose, cocoa, citric acid and ammonium – which speeds the nicotine 'hit' … [The Health Secretary] said that 'until very recently nobody knew about any of these ingredients', adding that he was demanding further information from the tobacco companies so that they could show which brands contained the additives.

The Times, 10 February 2000

NICOTINE FACTS:

- It only takes a maximum of 3 days for all of the nicotine to leave the body – no matter how many you smoke or for how long.
- Nicotine is the fastest-acting drug known to mankind.
- It only takes one single puff to get you hooked *if* you've been hooked before – no matter how long you've stopped for.
- Although it's most of the other chemicals in cigarettes which actually cause cancer, the only reason why people smoke is to get the powerful drug nicotine.
- Nicotine increases heart rate, increases blood pressure and constricts blood vessels.
- Nicotine patches and gums are a nonsensical way to try to stop smoking as they contain the very same drug that smokers are addicted to. This is the same as telling a heroin addict that instead of smoking it they should have it in a patch so they can get a gradual hit throughout the day!
- Despite the facts, there are more teenage girls smoking now than at any time in history.

The Six Essential Dietary Needs

The human body has six primary dietary needs, each as important as the other. A deficiency in any one of them can cause havoc to the intricate workings of the body so all are essential for amazing health.

Many traditionally trained dieticians and doctors will disagree with some of my suggestions as to the best sources of these dietary must-haves. This is often due to their unwillingness to stare common sense in the face, and also to the fact they are 'bound over' to teach traditional 'dietary law' in the way they were taught it.

One thing which is undisputed, however, is that it is essential we get a good supply of each of these 'human needs' on a daily basis for optimum health and vitality. It also cannot be disputed, although some try, that all of the foods meant for human consumption which come from the plant world contain, to some degree, all of the following six essential dietary needs.

Protein *Fat* Carbohydrate WATER Vitamins

Minerals Protein *Fat* Carbohydrate

Water Vitamins MINERALS **Protein** Fat

Carbohydrate *Water* Vitamins Minerals

Protein **Fat** Carbohydrate WATER Vitamins

Minerals Protein *Fat* Carbohydrate

Water **Vitamins** Minerals Protein *Fat*

Carbohydrate WATER Vitamins Minerals

Protein *Fat* Carbohydrate WATER Vitamins

Minerals Protein **Fat** Carbohydrate

Water Vitamins MINERALS Protein

Fat **Carbohydrate** Water Vitamins Minerals

Protein **FAT** Carbohydrate Water Vitamins

MINERALS **Protein** Fat Carbohydrate

Water **VITAMINS** PROTEIN **Fat**

Carbohydrate **Water** Vitamins Minerals

Protein *Fat* Carbohydrate WATER Vitamins

Minerals Protein *Fat* Carbohydrate

1. Protein

There has been a lot of hogwash over the years about how much protein we need and the best sources for the human body. Both the dairy industry and the meat industry – along with certain governments – have had vested interests in telling people that they will perish without plenty of animal protein. So successful has the propaganda been that the minute anyone even thinks of becoming a veggie, the first question people ask them is, 'But where on earth are you going to get your protein?' The fact is, however, no matter what you have read, heard or been brainwashed to believe, we can easily live without consuming any animal protein whatsoever.

This does not mean for one second that you will not gain *any* dietary benefit from eating fish, meat or cheese, as clearly you will. It just means that you can easily meet your protein needs by skipping all animal protein.

During the first six months of life, the average human being doubles in body weight. At no other time in our lives does this happen in such a short time span (although it can feel like it!). It is undisputed that we need more protein during that time and during the first few years of life than at any other time. It is also undisputed that the best food during that time is mother's milk. Mother's milk contains only 1.6 to 2.2 per cent protein, so why we need a beef steak which has over 20.3g of protein per 100g once we are adults and have stopped growing is a mystery to one and all.

Cows Don't Have Barbeques!

Some of the largest land animals are herbivores, consuming no meat, fish or dairy whatsoever. The elephant is perhaps the best example as it is by far the strongest and most muscular land animal. Hippos aren't exactly under-furnished in the muscle department either, nor are giraffes, rhinos, buffalo, deer and even cows. Not only do you never see them slapping a few burgers on the barbecue, but I shouldn't think you'll see them nipping to their local 'health' store to top up on their vitamin B12 either! These magnificent muscular land animals get *all* their protein needs from the vegetation which was designed specifically for them by Nature. Equally, humans can easily get their protein needs from eating fresh 'live' fruit, vegetation, nuts and seeds which were specifically designed for them.

Almonds contain almost as much protein as red meat and 6 per cent more calcium per 100g than plain yoghurt.

Amino Acids – the Building Blocks of Protein

In reality, we don't require any protein. What we actually need are amino acids, the building blocks of protein. The human body requires 23 amino acids. It can manufacture 15 all on its own but the other eight we must get from our diet. These are known as essential amino acids. All of these essential amino acids can be found in the plant kingdom, not just the animal kingdom. Avocados, once seen as the dieter's Kryptonite because of their fat content, are packed with all the essential amino acids. All fruits, vegetables, nuts and seeds contain plenty of these essential protein building blocks.

Getting a Healthy Balance

If you were thinking about going veggie (or vegan), please don't stress yourself about where you are going to get your protein from. As long as you have plenty of natural 'live' foods, Nature won't pay you back by making you ill with a protein deficiency. Equally, if you do eat fish, meat and some dairy, you will also be meeting your daily requirements for amino acids. However, you MUST also eat 'live' natural foods in order to keep the body trim and healthy. Personally, I eat plenty of cold-water fish, a *little* dairy sometimes and, given the choice between a plate of white refined pasta and some organic chicken, the meat would win most of the time.

The choice of whether you are vegan, veggie or what is considered 'normal' is up to you and all three can be very healthy as long as you follow a few rules. Equally, all three can be extremely detrimental to health if you go about it in the wrong way. If a vegan for example, stops eating animal products but simply replaces them with refined carbohydrates and little in the way of fresh fruit and vegetables, then they will actually be nutritionally worse off than if they ate some fish, chicken or 'live' yoghurt. And if a vegetarian stops eating meat only to replace it with loads of dairy, again they aren't doing themselves any favours on the health front. I have an extremely good friend who is vegan and who only went vegan for health reasons. However, although he never eats anything of animal origin, his food intake is far from the healthiest on the planet. He will turn down fish, chicken, eggs and so on, but is quite happy to tuck into a plate full of white bread (no butter clearly) and a bowl of white refined pasta. You will soon realize after the carbohydrate part in this section that you are much, much better off with some fish or chicken and some vegetables.

Best Protein Sources

Avocados

Broccoli

Kale

Spinach

Natural nuts – almonds, brazil, walnuts, etc.

Seeds – sunflower, pumpkin, sesame

Fish – sardines, tuna

Organic white meat

Tofu and all soya products

Organic white cheese

Quorn

Soya protein powder

Micro-filtered whey protein powder

'Live' cow's or goat's yoghurt

2. Fat

Never has one *essential* food had such bad press. The body needs fat. Without it we die – it's as simple as that. Yet most people still do anything to avoid it. If you get nothing else from this book you need to understand that YOU NEED TO EAT FAT!

Fat Lot of Good

Fat is as important to our diet as vitamins, minerals, carbohydrates and protein. It provides a concentrated source of energy and helps with the absorption and transportation of fat-soluble vitamins A, D, E and K. Fat is needed to maintain healthy skin and hair. It helps to regulate the appetite and to protect the organs. Fats are the basis of the body's steroid hormones, which control many functions including the central nervous system, sex and reproductive organs, cardiovascular and immune systems. Fats are also an important building material in cell membranes, helping to cover every nerve in the body and act as a good insulator.

In 1929, scientists Mildred and George Burr discovered the most important fats and oils in our diets – essential fatty acids (EFAs). The reason why they are called *essential* is because they cannot be manufactured in the body and *must* be eaten regularly in the forms of fats and oils.

Signs of Essential Fats Deficiency

Wounds not healing properly

Kidney failure

Liver degeneration

Breakdown of the immune system

Common infections

Skin problems

Hair loss

Dehydration

And an overall effect on most areas
    of your health

GOOD FATS
Don't Make You Fat!

Despite increased knowledge of the importance of 'good' fats, people still think they will pile on the pounds if they even look at an avocado! This, I believe, is mainly due to media dieticians telling us that 'fat contains more calories per gram than any other food group'. This nutritional fact led to the low-fat/high-carb diet mania of the 1980s and fuels the 'watch the fat' frenzy which is still very much alive today.

Even though carbohydrates contain less than half the number of calories of fat, we have become much fatter and unhealthier as a nation since we started swapping the fat for the carbs. This is because you don't need anywhere near as much fat before you have satisfied your appetite or, to be more accurate, your cravings!

A BBC *Horizon* documentary proved this point with research on the Atkins diet. They showed that despite a person being allowed to eat as much 'food' in the form of fat and protein as they wished on the Atkins diet, their calorie intake was *low*. This is because although they *could* eat and eat and eat, they didn't actually want to. They may well have had *mental* cravings for fries, cakes, bread and chocolate, as all those who have put themselves through the Atkins headache will testify, but, on a physical level, after a few days, they didn't actually feel hungry.

This is not just because fat helps to regulate appetite, but much more importantly because the body gets flushed of all drug-like foods and so all *unnatural physical* cravings, which feel like normal hunger, are eliminated. This is also why when people first go on programmes like the Atkins Diet the first few days are akin to a smoker stopping smoking. They seem to have a void which their new lifestyle cannot fill. Which is why, *at first*, they *do* eat more calories as they are trying to feed, what is essentially, a false hunger and trying hard to fill the void created by refined sugars and carbohydrates. Once the 'false hunger' has been starved, the physical void is no longer there and the amount of food they eat is *decreased*.

Fat is not an enemy – it's essential to your health and for helping to keep your hunger correctly balanced. Unfortunately, as you will have read in The Seven Deadly Dietary Sins (page 115), EFAs have been stripped from virtually all foods because of processing.

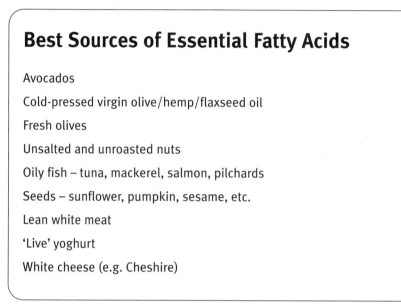

Best Sources of Essential Fatty Acids

Avocados

Cold-pressed virgin olive/hemp/flaxseed oil

Fresh olives

Unsalted and unroasted nuts

Oily fish – tuna, mackerel, salmon, pilchards

Seeds – sunflower, pumpkin, sesame, etc.

Lean white meat

'Live' yoghurt

White cheese (e.g. Cheshire)

3. Carbohydrate

Despite the popularity of low-carb diets, the fact remains that carbohydrates are a fundamental need for our health. Anyone embarking on a *completely* carbohydrate-free diet is risking some major health problems in the short and long term. However, like fat and protein, carbohydrates *must* come from the right sources to benefit health.

Unfortunately, when people think of carbohydrates, the first foods that spring to mind are 'man-made' as opposed to natural carbohydrates. In fact, whenever you see a list of carbohydrates, things like bread, pasta and other flour-based foods are often at the top. While these are carbohydrates, they are essentially man-made, meaning they have often been *heavily* processed in some way. Nature's finest form of carbohydrates – fruits and vegetables – need little, if any, processing. In fact, the less you process (cook) vegetables, the better most of them are for you. As for fruits, they were simply never designed with cooking in mind, not even 'cooking apples'!

It's Not All Black and White – More Brown and White

When you eat white bread and white pasta you are basically consuming a load of nutritionally poor junk. We have been told for years that pasta and bread are really good for us, but when they have been 'refined' to the extent of stripping virtually all vitamins, minerals and fibre from them, they end up being nothing more than fast-sugar-releasing junk food. Having said that, you still cannot be sure that brown man-made carbohydrates are good for you; food companies sometimes dye them with caramel to give the impression that they are 'good carbs'.

The ideal scenario is that virtually all your carbohydrates come from the natural sugars found in *all* fruits and vegetables. The truth is, despite what we are taught, we simply don't need any man-made carbs to live. *All* of our carbohydrate needs are found in abundance in the fresh fruits and vegetables we eat (or will be eating from now on!). So if you are eating plenty of freshly prepared salads, steamed or stir-fried veggies with some lean protein, you needn't think for one second you are on a no-carbs diet. In fact, you are consuming the best carbohydrates known to humankind.

When I say that all of our carbohydrate needs can be met through fruits and vegetables, I mean that all our *physical* carbohydrate needs can be met. Our mental needs are something else. In the real world, most people seem to need their daily fix of some kind of man-made carb. There is actually nothing wrong with this as many man-made carbs can still be nutritionally beneficial, as long as they haven't been too refined and they're not eaten in excess. The problem is, as you will have read in The Seven Deadly Dietary Sins (page 108), the more refined they are, the more likely they are to make you overeat.

There are four main man-made carbs, and here are my thoughts on each one:

Give Us This Day Our Daily Bread ... Or Not Perhaps!

Bread is probably the most addictive and problematic man-made carb. Most people would simply never even contemplate being without their daily dose. Many are under the terrible misapprehension that it's the best thing since, well, the sliced version of the stuff. However, your daily bread – even the healthy-looking wholemeal versions – is often a far cry from the healthiest thing you can put into your body.

Your average innocent-looking loaf contains all sorts of dietary nightmares: yeast, salt, sugar, anti-fungals, saturated fats, hydrogenated fats, wheat and many more. Now you may think it's fair to say that sugar, salt and refined fats are no-nos when it comes to health but wheat is perfectly natural. Wheat may have had good publicity from the people responsible for harvesting and selling the stuff, but it's far from what the human body had in mind.

Wheat is the single largest contributor to intestinal dysbiosis, parasitic infections and universal food allergies. As with smoking, the body can take in foreign invaders for years before we start to notice any real problems. Consuming too much wheat has been linked to fatigue, memory loss, sleep disruption, muscle and joint pain, high blood pressure, asthma, headaches, visual disturbances, learning difficulties, constipation, and inability to absorb vital nutrients – to name just a few.

As you can imagine, wheat doesn't feature in the 14-day Turbo-charge Your Life programme, but this doesn't mean you should *never* eat anything with wheat in it again. It's just that when you have experienced two weeks free of wheat *and* refined man-made carbs, you won't want to go back to them on a regular basis. There's nothing wrong with having some wholemeal bread every now and then, but if you can kick it altogether you will be doing yourself a massive favour on the weight, health and energy front.

Just because you go wheat-free doesn't mean you have to go without bread. There are all sorts of wonderful breads on the market these days which don't contain any wheat, sugar, salt or refined fats; most have slow-releasing sugars and are extremely satisfying. These include breads made from rye, spelt, pumpernickel, quinoa and more, all of which are in a different league to wheat-based bog-standard loaves.

Rice

Of all the 'man-made' carbs out there, rice is the one exception. The Japanese have proved that eating rice causes neither weight problems nor premature death. In fact, with the Japanese living longer than any other race, it would perhaps prove the opposite to be true.

Again, I think relying on your gut instinct is the best bet. Often if I eat pasta I feel bloated and tired, yet the same rarely, if ever, happens when I eat rice. Rice only has to be steamed to be eaten and is an excellent source of fibre, vitamins and minerals. When buying rice, look for rice as close to its original state as possible, such as wild rice, wholegrain rice or even basmati rice, and keep clear of the white refined versions.

Pasta

Most of the pasta we eat is of the white, refined variety. Refining and bleaching destroys at least 70 per cent of its vitamin content and up to 90 per cent of its mineral content. White flour is also pretty devoid of fibre, meaning it will raise blood-sugar levels quickly. It also contains inorganic iron, which depletes other good vitamins.

Pasta can cause incredible dehydration and stomach bloating immediately after eating it. Although said to provide energy, eating a big bowl of it often has an extremely soporific effect, leaving you feeling tired and lethargic.

Pasta doesn't feature anywhere during the 14-day Turbo-charge Your Life programme, and you will feel so much better for it. This doesn't mean, however, that you should never have it again. I would say, though, that you may well want to skip white pasta for the rest of your life, although trying to get wholegrain pasta in a restaurant is pretty tricky to say the least. Look for wholegrain/wholemeal versions or get hold of pasta which isn't made with wheat, such as hemp or spelt pasta, and always make a point of eating this sort of pasta with a salad.

Potatoes

The French have always said, 'Potatoes are for pigs and corn is for cattle.' Why? Because they help to fatten them up!

Baked potatoes have always been seen as a health food and often as an aid to slimming. I know many people who are careful not to add butter to their jacket potatoes, but have no problem eating the potato itself. What they don't realize is that it's the white potato that is fattening, not so much the butter. You will notice that I have said *white* potato. Like all carbohydrates, white versions are the worst for you on a health and fat level. I'm not saying that a baked white potato is as bad as white pasta, but you must understand that even though it appears natural, it is still classed as a manmade carbohydrate because it has been heavily processed (cooked).

You will notice in the recipes that I have not used white potatoes, but sweet potatoes. Sweet potatoes will not cause the same 'fast sugar' response as baked white potatoes. If you are going to have white potatoes, then make sure they are boiled, not baked, and certainly make sure they're not fried!

Personally I must say I love white potatoes, baked and boiled, and when you are on the second phase of your life programme, i.e. after the 14 days, you will no doubt tuck into them every now and then. There's nothing wrong with this – *at times* – but please do not delude yourself into thinking they are the best slimming and health food on the planet because they are a far cry from that.

Best Sources of Carbohydrate in Order

Vegetables – *all* except white potatoes

Vegetable juices – green ones are best mixed with carrot or apple

Whole fruits

Wild/brown/basmati rice

Breads – spelt, rye, hemp, pumpernickel, but NOT WHEAT!

Pasta – hemp, spelt, rice, or wholemeal durum wheat if nothing else

Wholemeal pitta – the only wheat-based bread on this list, but use
   very sparingly!

4. Water

Never underestimate the power of water. It is vital for optimum health. It provides the environment in which the body's chemical reactions take place, and the solution in which the food we eat is dissolved and transported.

You can go for months without food, but only days without water. It is essential we get enough of this super liquid fuel *daily*. This does *not*, however, necessarily mean you have to drink 2 litres, or 8 glasses, of water a day to meet your needs. One of the reasons we need to drink so much water is because the vast majority of what we eat and drink these days has not only been stripped of its natural water content but actually causes dehydration.

The vast majority of foods which were designed specifically for the human body – ripe fruits and fresh vegetables – *all* contain a high percentage of water. A watermelon is over 95 per cent water, and even a banana contains over 80 per cent of life's essential fluid.

Because most of what the average Brit consumes on the SUK (Standard UK) diet causes dehydration – salt, alcohol, bread, soft drinks, man-made carbohydrates, sugar – the signals to the brain get distorted. When your cells are starved of water, the body sends signals to the brain calling for some. When this happens it is natural for the brain to receive a *hunger* signal rather than one for thirst. This is because Nature's foods are full of water, and when we first started life on this planet you couldn't exactly nip to your nearest corner shop to get a bottle of Evian, nor indeed could you just turn on a tap. Water, as we know it today, wasn't readily available, and this is precisely why Nature made sure that if we consumed the foods she provided for us we would not suffer from hunger *or* dehydration.

Water on Tap – or Perhaps Not

Water is the fastest-growing sector of the 'soft-drinks' industry. Bottled water is now worth £1.5 billon in the UK alone. When water first started to be bottled, the vast majority of people thought it would never take off; after all, who would pay for bottled water when you could get it from a tap? When I used to go abroad as a child I thought it was crazy that you couldn't drink the water from the tap and had to get it from a bottle. If my uncle George from Yorkshire were still alive today he would take one look at everyone drinking bottled water in the UK and think the world had gone mad. However, it's not as mad as he may have thought. If he got wind of what was in the average supply of tap water, he might well have joined the bottled water revolution.

This is not to say that tap water in the UK is poison, or that it won't sustain life, or that it's worse than soft drinks which are full of chemicals and sugar. All I'm saying is that some of the chemicals found in our tap water aren't all they're cracked up to be.

The best quality water is that found in organically grown raw fruits and vegetables. You can access the amazing combination of water and 'live' nutrients either by eating them or extracting the juice from them. But in terms of straightforward drinking water, the jury is still very much out on which one is best. Look out for the words 'spring' and 'mineral' on labels. Mineral water is natural water which has been filtered by the mountains and bottled at source. Spring water, however, can come from pretty much anywhere – including your tap! You will find, for example, that own-brand waters found in many gym chains are basically filtered tap water. Filtered water is clearly better than tap water as some of the nasties are filtered out, but it's worth knowing that not all filters are the same and in many cases chemicals like fluoride still remain.

Your best bet is to buy *any* bottled 'mineral' water as a supplement to the water in your foods and freshly extracted juices. The recommended daily water intake is 2 litres, but please bear in mind that this is for someone who hardly consumes any water-rich foods, and it doesn't take into account the weather or exercise levels.

The best quality water is that found in organically grown raw fruits and vegetables. You can access the amazing combination of water and 'live' nutrients either by eating them or extracting the juice from them.

5. Vitamins

With the explosion of vitamin supplements over the past 20 years, it makes you wonder how we ever got by without them. The vitamin-supplement market is now worth millions: in the UK alone we spend £300–400 million a year on these over-the-counter apparent health boosters. I say *apparent* because there is still no concrete proof that they have any benefits whatsoever. In fact, overloading the body with a pile of synthetic vitamins in a desperate attempt to make up for a poor diet has been shown to be harmful.

Overdosing on synthetic vitamins has even caused deaths!

When it comes to vitamins, recommended amounts vary widely. EU guidelines are much higher than the UK's RDA (recommended daily allowance), and much of the research into vitamins involves far higher amounts. The body will often see these synthetic vitamins as foreign invaders and flush them out. If you think about the amount of money being spent on these things, that's pretty expensive wee!

There's no disputing the fact that vitamins are an essential part of our diet. This was shown clearly in the 16th and 17th centuries when thousands of sailors died of scurvy due to a lack of vitamin C. We now know that deficiency in certain vitamins leads directly to disease.

Once again, Nature didn't forget to include vitamins in the foods she recommended for us. Every single fruit, vegetable, grain, nut and seed contains many thousands of vitamins, all in their natural state; all in a form which can be used by the human body; and all in exactly the right dose.

If you do need more vitamins, 99.9 per cent of the time it is because you are not getting them in your diet. Therefore by far the best way to remedy the situation is not to take a pill, which contains only one section of Nature's nutritional jigsaw puzzle, but to meet those needs through 'live' foods and freshly extracted juices, both of which will supply you with the right amounts of vitamins you need.

6. Minerals

Just like vitamins, the market for synthetic mineral supplements is booming. The message is clear: if you aren't eating enough fruit and veg, just pop a pill or two and all will be fine and dandy. But you cannot live on vitamin and mineral pills.

You need to get as many minerals as possible from the foods and juices you consume. It is much easier for the body to absorb minerals from food and freshly extracted juices than it is from a pill.

Modern farming methods, including the use of chemical pesticides, have affected the amount of minerals, such as zinc and selenium, in even the most 'natural' foods available to us. With that in mind, synthetic minerals can be of benefit in *some* cases of genuine mineral deficiency, but overall you cannot beat the real thing. Choose organic fruit and veg where possible.

Minerals can only be taken into our bodies in food. None can be manufactured by the body, as can some vitamins, so we must obtain all the minerals we need from food. Not all minerals are healthy, such as mercury and lead, and we do ingest both friendly and unfriendly ones. Plants and other animals which provide our food are equally harmed by toxic minerals, and they filter out much of the harmful minerals for us, so we ingest a much smaller amount.

Minerals are very stable, but can be lost through cooking, so juicing is ideal.

Common Foods Which Fit into the Six Essential Dietary Human Needs

All vegetables except jacket potatoes (raw, steamed, stir-fried, lightly boiled)

Balsamic vinegar

Beans – lentils, soya, mung, etc.

Breads – rye, spelt, quinoa, millet, wheat-/yeast-free, wholemeal pittas, good quality wholegrain with as few additives as possible

Butter – organic 'slightly salted' or no salt

Cheese – organic white – Cheshire is the best choice

Cold-pressed oils – olive, hemp, etc.

Dried fruit – must be eaten sparingly as can cause sugar levels to rise too rapidly. Non-sulphured apricots are the best choice.

Eggs – only free-range and organic

Fish – organic where possible

Fresh herbs – tarragon, thyme, mint, dill, fennel, ginger, cinnamon, oregano, rosemary, bay, etc.

Fruit juices – *only* freshly extracted. *Always* drink slowly and diluted with ice or water to prevent a sudden surge in sugar levels, and have no more than a couple of glasses a day.

Fruit smoothies – whole fruits blended with freshly extracted fruit juice and/or live yogurt. As these are energy-dense drinks, you need to use sparingly or as an aid for working out or weight-training.

Herbal teas – camomile, fennel, peppermint, lemon, ginger, nettle, red-clover, etc.

Honey – must be raw or Manuka 'active'. Virtually all other honey is just like sugar!

Lamb – the only 'red' meat that fits into this category

'Live' yoghurt – with no artificial sweeteners or refined sugar (Rachel's Organic with Honey or Vanilla are just lovely or get a plain live yoghurt and add fresh berries – beautiful)

Milk – non-sweetened soya milk, or if you are using sparingly, semi-skimmed organic milk

Mineral water

Nut butters

Nuts and seeds – non-roasted and non-salted – almonds, brazil nuts, cashews, walnuts, hazelnuts, pecans, pistachios, pumpkin, sesame, sunflower, flax, etc.

Pastas – hemp, spelt, wholegrain

Potatoes – white boiled or sweet

Rice – wild/brown/basmati – best choice of all processed carbohydrates

Sea vegetables – nori, sea palm, dulse, kelp

Sprouts

Sushi – vegetarian or regular

Vegetable juices – mixed with apple/carrot/pineapple juice to taste

Veggie stuff – tofu, Quorn, soya, etc.

Wheatgrass juice

White meat – good quality and organic where possible

Whole fruits

Whole rolled oats

Wine and Champagne – organic white and red (use your common sense on amounts!)

Seeing Is Believing

Or should that be believing is seeing? Whatever your goals, you stand a much better chance of making them happen when you see the results in advance. And the only way to do this is using the power of the mind.

Visualization may seem slightly American or, quite frankly, weird as hell, but there's no question that when your brain sees what it wants in advance and stays focused on that image, you stand a much better chance of the thing you want actually materializing.

One amazing example of this is cyclist Bradley Wiggins. Bradley won a gold medal in the men's 4 km individual pursuit at the 2004 Olympic Games, something he predicted he would do when he was just 12. He says: 'This gold medal is something I've wanted to do since I was 12 years old, watching Chris Boardman win gold in Barcelona. I decided then that I really wanted to win Olympic gold.' And deciding, not *hoping*, is the key here.

Not only did he decide by voicing it to himself, but he wrote clearly that day in his diary that he would win Olympic Gold in that event. Not only did he write down that he would win Olympic Gold, but he even stated the year – 2004. He did enter the event at the Olympics in the year 2000 but he *only* got silver!

This is an incredible example of what can happen when you make a decision and do whatever it takes to achieve it. This is helped considerably by setting a date and visualizing what you want on a daily, if not weekly basis.

Jonny Wilkinson, the magnificent English rugby player, practised kicking that ball through the posts over and over again. He also visualized over and over again kicking the winning goal for his country in a World Cup final, something he achieved with the last kick of the game in the 2003 World Cup final in Australia.

Whether you believe it or not, there is no question that when you visualize your goals on a daily basis your brain, on both a conscious and subconscious level, will automatically make choices that will bring you closer to that goal.

With that in mind, whatever your goals on a physical level, get a crystal clear picture of how you want to look and feel in the future and focus with your eyes closed on that image for a few minutes every morning and a few minutes every night. The idea is to make the picture as clear and as bright as you can. You should imagine what it would be like living your life in that light, energy-driven body. Picture yourself clearly in clothes you would love to look good in; imagine what it's like to be able to breathe easily and have vibrant energy; see and feel exactly what you will be like in the future. If you do this properly, you will find that you can't help but get excited, and it's when this happens, when you get 'fully associated' with the picture, that your brain will do everything within its power to make sure you achieve it. That picture will then be with you when you are working out or making certain food choices. Visualization is an extremely powerful tool and, even if you don't necessarily believe in it, what harm is there in giving it a go for just 14 days?

Remember, this is a 14-day programme designed to create momentum for life. I fully believe that anyone can do anything for 14 days – if they are committed!

The next 14 days, if properly applied, can change every single aspect of your life, and especially your health, shape and energy levels. You have probably been itching to get cracking for some time, so without further ado, let's make a start …

The Turbo-charge Your Life in 14 Days Programme

Those Who Fail to Prepare – Prepare to Fail

In order for this programme to work you need to be prepared both mentally and on a practical level. I live in the real world, and you and I know that all the best intentions can easily go out of the window unless things are to hand. I know, for example, that if I forget to stockpile fruits, vegetables, fish, whole grains and other foods for my six essential dietary needs, I am less likely to eat well; and unless I'm prepared for my morning workout the night before, it's all too easy to hit that snooze button and turn over again. When it comes to the next 14 life-changing days, it is imperative that you are fully prepared *before* you start. Get what you need, set a date, stick to it and Turbo-charge Your Life!

What You Will Need for the Next 14 Days – *and Beyond!*

▪ The Right, Grateful and Inspired Mental Attitude

You should have this attitude by now. If you need a refresher, please re-read 'Ditch the Diets' (page 78).

▪ An Excellent Supply of Good-quality Fresh Vegetables and Selected Fruits

This is essential to the programme as you will be making lots of fresh juices and tasty recipes over the next 14 days. See the list of fruit and veg on page 257.

▪ An Excellent Supply of Good-quality Foods from the Six Dietary Needs List (page 157)

As well as vegetables and fruits, you will also need a good supply of other foods, such as lean meats, fish, wild rice and Quorn.

▪ A Juice Extractor

Not all juice extractors are built the same and you will need one that can take the job on for *your* needs. There are many different aspects to consider when buying a juicer: price; how many you're juicing for on a daily basis; what you need it for (general health, serious health, weight loss etc.); how it looks in your kitchen (as you should never show it the cupboard!) and so on. With that in mind it is important to know before investing in a machine that you are getting the right one. Our team is always on hand to answer your juicing needs *before* you buy. It is all to easy to just go and buy one, but you may well spend more than you need to or not enough for your needs. Call our juicy hotline on 0845 1 30 28 29 or visit www.thejuicemaster.com

■ A Blender

Most people already own one, but any blender will do the job.

■ A Personal Stereo of Some Kind

This is a great tool for your workouts. Although it's not essential, exercising to your favourite music really does make a difference.

■ A Mini-trampoline

Again this is not essential and you can choose your own form of exercise, but I'm a huge fan. Other than swimming, trampolining is the only cardiovascular exercise that works every muscle without jarring the joints. Not all mini-trampolines are built the same, so visit www.juicemaster.com for advice. Other exercise options are joining a gym or getting some running gear or rollerblades. Whatever you choose, just get moving!

■ A Flask

You will need this for taking juices and soups to work.

■ A Good Alarm Clock!

A VERY important piece of kit for this programme. For 14 days, at least, you will be kick-starting your day earlier than normal as you need time to work out and make your juice.

The Rules for the Next 14 Days

■ No White Flour Whatsoever

This should not only be a rule for the 14-day programme but also for life – as you will have read by now (see Chapter 7).

■ No Food with Wheat or Yeast

This rule is vital on a weight and energy level. You don't even need to know the 'why' behind it; all you need to know is that if you leave these out of the diet you will feel an incredible difference, especially to your energy levels.

■ No Picking between Meals

Self-explanatory really, but one of the habits we are looking to get into is letting hunger build and then getting incredible pleasure from truly satisfying that hunger with beautiful foods.

■ Chew Your Food Thoroughly

This is a very important part of the programme. Your stomach doesn't have teeth and struggles when large lumps of food come in without being properly masticated. Even the Turbo Smoothies, although in a liquid form, should be 'chewed' first – swill them around your mouth and take your time with them. Mixing food with saliva is essential for proper digestion. One of the biggest causes of overweight is the 'shovel it in as quick as I can' mentality. It seems bizarre that the same people who say they can't do without this food or that food because of the taste are the same people who never actually have the food in their mouth for long enough to taste it! Of all the things I teach, chewing your food thoroughly, eating slowly, whatever that food is, is the single most important thing you can do for long-term weight loss.

Have as Much as You Like – within Reason!

As long as you heed the previous rule you are welcome to eat as much as you like, until you are comfortably full. This programme isn't about portion sizes; it's more about eating the right fuel and in the right way. What a person does physically, their size, their shape, etc. will determine how much 'fuel' they require. So clearly it's never a case of one 'portion' size fits all. However, it is essential that you only ever eat when you are genuinely hungry and STOP EATING WHEN YOU ARE COMFORTABLY FULL. You will notice that some of the juice/smoothie/soup and whole-food recipes may well make more than your 'fuel' requirements at that time; if that's the case simply STOP EATING AT THE POINT YOU ARE FULL AND LEAVE THE REST. One woman I spoke to said, 'I love the morning Turbo Smoothie but sometimes I find it hard to finish it and I have to force it down.' Please, whatever you do, NEVER FORCE ANYTHING DOWN. The old adage of 'less is more' certainly applies here. You will not do your body more good by forcing anything down, even if it's good. Only eat when you are hungry and stop eating when you start to feel full. I know it's a concept which eludes most people, but you don't actually have to clear your plate or finish what's in your glass. I know we were told for years by our guardians that we should as 'there are starving people in Africa', but I think we have long since realized that us getting fat and ill by eating everything on our plates does nothing to help anyone in the world with a food shortage!

No 'Man-made' Carbs after 6pm (Potatoes, Rice, Pasta and Bread)

This is an amazing yet simple tool for weight-loss. Beyond the 14 days, it can be used for life to *stay* in the land of the slim, trim and healthy. Although it will feel slightly weird at first, once you get used to how light you feel in the evenings, you will love it. One of the main reasons for this rule is to make sure that when you exercise on an empty stomach the following morning you will be tapping into your *fat* stores rather than sugar stores. This aids weight-loss and makes you feel much less sluggish in the evening.

After the 14-day programme, the only starchy carb I would suggest in the evening is brown or wild rice. It's not as heavy as pasta and is a very good source of fibre. This doesn't mean you should never have carbs again in the evening. It just means that if you want to lose weight and get the body of your dreams, it's worth making it a rule *most* of the time.

■ Exercise Twice a Day for 30–60 Minutes

The Turbo-charge Your Life Programme does precisely that. This means we are not going to pussyfoot around with one hour of exercise three times a week – we will be exercising for one hour TWICE a day! This doesn't mean you need to pound your body to the point of damaging yourself – PLEASE, PLEASE, PLEASE whatever you do ALWAYS use your common sense. Many of you will be starting exercise for the first time in years and after the first day you will ache in places you didn't even know existed, so don't go so far that you sense you may hurt yourself. Equally though, don't make excuses and take it too easy. The idea is to get up and move your ass in some way for 30–60 minutes *twice* a day for 13 of the 14 days – please take one day off on the exercise front to give the body time to rest.

The exercise you choose doesn't have to be high impact and for some just walking will be a major feat. The exercise can be anything; aerobic classes, trampolining, swimming, yoga, running, stretching, weight-training, walking or a combination. I rarely, for example, jump on my trampoline for more than half an hour, so I often do press-ups, sit-ups and a little breathing and stretching to fill the other half an hour. If you find one hour is just too much, you must at least do 30 minutes of serious exercise – to the point where you sweat!

■ Visualize Your Goals Every Morning *and* Every Night

This may seem strange, but seeing really is believing. If you get a clear picture of how you want to look and feel in the future, and make it as real in your mind's eye as you can, you brain is more likely to make decisions

Ask Yourself the Following Questions on Waking

What am I grateful for today?
Who am I grateful for today?
What can I do today to make it special?

I realize how silly those questions can sound, but it's a damn sight better than waking up bitching or worrying about 'stuff'. You can change the questions as you wish, to things like 'What is good in my life at the moment?' but one of the key mental tools I want to teach is living with a degree of gratitude. When you begin to feel grateful, your life immediately feels more fulfilled. If your brain can't find an answer to your questions then simply add 'what could' at the beginning. For example, instead of 'What am I grateful for?' ask 'What could I be grateful for if I really thought about it?' Don't just ask the question without allowing your brain to search for an answer!

that day which will take you closer to your goal. Like all of the 'rules', even if it feels silly, just do it!

■ Drink 2 Litres of Water Every Day

Although you will be eating plenty of hydrating meals and drinking plenty of freshly extracted juice, it's worth drinking a couple of litres of water a day to help the body shift unwanted toxins. For the best type of water, see page 153.

■ Spend No More than 2 Hours on Recreational TV and Computer Use Each Day

If you can get rid of the TV altogether for the next 14 days, that will drastically change your life. Such drastic measures aren't essential but a curb on your couch-potato activities is a must. If you are going to do something then do it properly, and doing this programme properly means 'turning off the TV to go do something less boring instead'.

No Eating for 3 Hours before Bed

This is crucial as when you sleep your metabolism slows down. Having to digest food means your body is still working when it should be resting. Eating late at night also contributes to what can only be described as a 'food hangover', making getting up difficult and working out even more so. Having said this, if you find that doing your evening workout means you are eating 1 or 2 hours before bed time, that's perfectly OK. When you exercise your basal metabolic rate remains faster a few hours afterwards. It is also much better to eat than not to if you are genuinely hungry, even if it's an hour before bed. Where possible, do not eat *just* before you sleep. If you are hungry just before sleep you will find a glass of water usually does the trick.

Don't Allow Your Thoughts to Revolve around the Programme

This programme is designed to Turbo-charge Your Life – not become your life! When people embark on programmes, their whole life often becomes all about the next meal! Yes, it will be weird at first, and yes, you need to prepare, but don't forget to live. Remember, this isn't a diet – it's a system designed to change your lifestyle.

Follow Each Day to the Letter

The programme is rather like a good recipe – if you don't follow it correctly you will not get the same results. Everything in the plan is here for a reason, and you need to look at each one like an ingredient. Miss just one and you'll get a very different end result. The key is not to look for any 'buts' and, for once, just get on with it!

Things to Know before You Start

◼ You Will Lose Weight

If you follow this programme to the letter – *and you are overweight* – you will lose inches and 8–14 lb over the next 14 days. If you are a woman, you will drop at least a dress size.

◼ You May Not Feel Well

You may experience some headaches and a dip in energy over the first three to four days, and you may get some spots! This is nothing to worry about. It is simply your body 'cleaning the house' and changing from sugar-burning to fat-burning. If you find you want to go to bed much earlier than usual, that's perfectly fine and normal.

◼ Breakfast Doesn't Change Much over the 14 Days

This is because The Juice Master's Turbo-charge Smoothie contains everything the body needs to sustain energy and 'clean the house' at the same time.

◼ You May Feel Hungrier than Usual for the First 3–4 Days

This is perfectly normal. It is caused by the 'sugar parasites' asking for their usual fix and is a false hunger – one which usually keeps people deluded and hooked! The beauty is that you will have sufficiently starved them after a few days. You'll find they stop calling and your sugar levels will return to how they should be.

It is easy to mistake emotion for hunger. Always ask yourself before you eat, 'Am I genuinely hungry, or am I bored/stressed/lonely/upset/in need of a reward, etc.?' A good question to ask is, 'On a scale from 1 to 10, how hungry am I?' If you feel about a number 4, then you aren't really hungry. You are aiming to eat when you feel between level 7 and

8. If you reach level 10, you have left it too long and you could end up eating anything!

■ Be Prepared to Experience Increased Energy

After the first four or five days your energy levels may increase to the point where you find yourself sleeping less. This is all good, but sometimes people don't know what to do with their new-found energy and time. Again, preparation is key. Buy some books, think of a new hobby or channel that energy into a new business venture which really could change your life.

■ The First Five Days are the Cleaning Part of the Programme

You will notice that your food intake will probably be less than you're used to. However, the *quality* of nutrition will be much higher so, on a cellular level, your body will actually be getting more nutrients than usual. As mentioned, you may feel hungrier and even more tired during the first few days, but that is not due to a lack of food; it is purely down to 'withdrawal' symptoms from the drug-like foods and drinks. It is imperative that you stick to the menu choices available, or your own variation that follows the principles. For example, if the recipe is for tuna and avocado and lemon juice all mixed together and you want mackerel or sardines etc. – then change the recipe. You are also welcome to add grated, shredded or diced vegetables (cucumber, carrot, peppers etc.) to this kind of recipe. Equally, if you find one particular recipe works for you and you want to have it every day – feel free!

■ Start on a Monday!

I have designed the programme to be started on a Monday. This is because the weekends are 'different' in people's heads and, in the real world, our eating and drinking choices change slightly (or a lot) during the weekends. This doesn't mean you have to start on this day; if it suits you better, start on any day you like – it will be just as effective.

■ Get Plenty of Rest

Sleep is a vital component of the cleansing part of the programme, particularly during the first five days. Unfortunately, it has become almost uncool to sleep, but trust me – in order for you to remain focused on your goal and be bright as a button in the morning, you are aiming for at least six to eight hours of sleep. If that means hitting the sack at 9 p.m., then do it. Whatever you think of him, George W Bush has a rule of being in bed by 9.30 p.m. and rarely does he break it. Rest is paramount for Turbo-charging Your Life and getting a turbo-start each morning during the programme.

■ If You Want to Have the Turbo-charge Smoothie for Breakfast *and* Lunch – Feel Free

Many people who have done this programme have said they found it very easy to just make more of the Turbo-charge Smoothie in the morning, pour half in a flask, stick it in the fridge and have it for lunch as well.

■ If You Feel Like You Need More Food – EAT!

If you find that you feel hungry late afternoon then eat! What many people do is either keep a good supply of the Green Power Veggie Soup to dip into or they make up a big bowl of the JM Snack Attack, add some grated veggies to it and tuck in when they get a bit peckish. However, please make sure you ONLY eat when you are genuinely hungry and do not to try to fill a gap in your day or your life.

■ The Turbo-charge Smoothie Makes More Than Is Needed For One Person

The Turbo-charge Smoothie makes about 1 litre of juice. This is normally too much for the average person, but fine for some. As mentioned, never force it down and only consume enough for your needs. Always pour the excess into a flask and have as a 'snack' throughout the day.

Just to reiterate, never eat or drink more than is comfortable – even if it's good food!

■ It's Only 14 Days!

Although the programme lasts for only 14 days, it is a launch pad which will have a wonderful knock-on effect on every single part of your life. However, it is essential that you complete the 14 days without any slip-ups. For once, you don't want to hear yourself saying, 'But this happened or that happened.' One thing about life is that 'shit happens', and I can guarantee that you will never find a hassle-free 14-day period in your life. People use these 'moments' as excuses, but let's get this clear: 'unless you look after your body you'll have nowhere to live' – so nothing is more important than this.

Stay 100 per cent focused and do whatever it takes to complete the 14 days.

If you have any 'moments' when you feel you can't be bothered then please, before you do anything else, have a shower or bath and reread 'No More Excuses' (page 6).

Days 1 to 5 (Monday to Friday)

Morning

- Get up in plenty of time for your morning workout.
- Drink a glass of water before you do anything else, preferably warm water with lemon or lime.
- Spend a few minutes deep breathing, asking your three questions (page 167) and doing your visualization (page 159–60). **THIS IS IMPORTANT!**
- Put on your gym/walking clothes and head to the park/gym or wherever you are choosing to do your morning physical wake-up.
- Put music on and begin your morning workout of 45–60 minutes.
- Make The Juice Master's Turbo-charge Smoothie (page 195) and prepare lunch if it needs preparing in advance. If you are going straight to the gym, make your smoothie before you go, seal it in a flask and ask the people at the gym to leave it in their fridge. You can then drink it slowly in the sauna or when you come out.

Lunch

- Get oxygen circulating as often as possible by doing some deep-breathing exercises. Do some more visualization, as the more your brain sees the direction it wants to go in, the more likely it is to get there. If you have time, do some sort of very light exercise. No matter how busy we are at work we can usually find at least 10 minutes to go for a walk before lunch. Personally, I have a mini-trampoline in the office, and when I feel sluggish I hop on it for a few minutes and boom! – back to normal.
- Choose any one of The Juice Master's Turbo lunches overleaf.

Lunch Options

■ Choose from the first three options for the first five days. If, however, you start getting too hungry and feel yourself slipping into 'diet' mentality then go for the other options. Having said that, you will be amazed at just how filling the first three options are.

▲ The Juice Master's Turbo Salad – Light Version (page 213)

▲ Green Veggie Power Soup (page 219) – Best to make the night before, heat in the morning and put in a flask ready for lunch. The recipe makes enough for four so you'll have some for another day or so.

▲ The Juice Master's Protein Snack Attack (page 229)

▲ 1 tub Rachel's Organic Live Yogurt with Honey (available in supermarkets)

▲ Jasey's Veggie Sushi Rolls (page 226) – just beautiful!

After Work – Late Afternoon/Early Evening

This is an ideal time to have your second *main* workout of the day. Clearly, if it isn't the best time for you then don't 'but' – just find a way around it and have your workout later. Jump on your mini-trampoline; go for a run with your headphones on; head to the gym; play a game of rounders or football; put your rollerblades on; do an hour of yoga; or simply go for a long walk. Whatever you do, though, you must do it until you sweat. Many people 'stroll' around the park and believe they are getting as good a workout as those who are working up a sweat – well they're not! If you are going to walk, walk *fast* and get your heart pumping!

For the first two days, you should ideally have a 'natural' dinner containing 100 per cent 'live', natural foods, such as a main-course salad, soup or a turbo-style veggie smoothie. If, however, you really are hungry like the proverbial wolf, then I have included other options. Please choose from the following:

Dinner Options

- ▲ The Juice Master's Turbo Salad – Main Course Version (page 214)
- ▲ Green Veggie Power Soup or any soup from the soup section (pages 218–22)
- ▼ Jasey's Fish Kebabs with Pineapple and Steamed Veggies (page 236)
- ▼ Honey-glazed Vegetables (page 235)
- ▼ Oven-steamed Chicken and Vegetables (page 234)
- ▼ Thyme for Tuna (page 233)
- ▼ Alternatively, you are free to use any of your own recipes that consist of a protein-based meal (fish/chicken/tofu/Quorn) with plenty of salad and/or stir-fried veggies. This combination gives you an immense choice.

- ▦ Do a 10-minute visualization of your goals while breathing deeply and listening to relaxing music.
- ▦ Do not eat anything else before you sleep but keep drinking plenty of water, herbal teas or hot water with lemon or lime.
- ▦ Get to bed. You want to be up early tomorrow!

the programme

Days 6 and 7 (Saturday and Sunday)

It's the weekend – so watch out!

One common pattern is being 'good' during the week and bingeing at weekends. This is why days six and seven are so important in terms of breaking old patterns of behaviour. It is essential you stay focused during the next two days and remain committed to doing whatever it takes to complete the programme.

If you decided to go for the 'pure natural' meal options during the past five days, not only will you have had the best results, but the introduction of some good-quality processed foods will be very welcome at this stage. On a food level, the rules for these two days couldn't be simpler. You will be having a Turbo-charge Smoothie for breakfast, a light carbohydrate-based lunch and a protein-rich dinner – not rocket science.

The best option is to stay clear of *all* man-made carbs for the entire 14-day programme. However, if doing so would be too tricky for *you* or would make you slip into 'diet' mentality, then I would much rather you had them. Just make sure they're from the 'lunch option' menu in this section as these are good-quality carbs that release sugar slowly and will not interfere with your success. As for the first five days, though, if you are quite happy having one of the first three 'natural' options on the lunch menu then feel free – by the time you reach the end of the 14 days you will be glad you did.

Many people get into the routine of having a Turbo-charge Smoothie for breakfast *and* lunch, and a protein-rich dinner. If you choose this approach, it will have the most dramatic results in terms of weight loss and health. It also means you can make your lunch at the same time as breakfast. And it's a no-brainer to follow.

Morning

- Get up in plenty of time for your morning workout and to make a Turbo-charge Smoothie (page 195).
- Drink a glass of water before you do anything else, preferably warm water with lemon or lime.
- Spend a few minutes breathing deeply, asking your three questions (page 167) and doing your visualization (pages 159–60). **THIS IS IMPORTANT!**
- Put on your gym/walking clothes and head to the park/gym or wherever you are choosing to do your morning physical wake-up.
- Put music on and begin your morning workout of 45–60 minutes.
- Make a Turbo-charge Smoothie or Turbo-charge Weekend Breakfast Smoothie (page 200) Although we are looking to get into a similar pattern of eating behaviour at weekends as during the week, I acknowledge that a fruit-based smoothie would be most welcome at this juncture, which is why I have included the Weekend Breakfast Smoothie.

NOTE: If you are waking up and going straight to the gym, make your smoothie before you go, seal it in a flask and ask the people at the gym to leave it in their fridge. You can then drink it in the sauna or when you come out.

Lunch

- As it's the weekend, chances are you'll have more time during the day to get your body moving! Remember you are looking to create a new pattern of behaviour over the 14 days and to move your body as much as possible. Once again, this doesn't mean battering yourself; it just means taking time to go for a long walk, do some deep-breathing or, if you are reasonably healthy, increasing your exercise at weekends.
- Prepare/have lunch from the following menus choices:

Lunch Options

▲ The Juice Master's Green Power Smoothie (page 196) – Again, this can be made in advance when you are making your morning Turbo-charge Smoothie. If you prefer, you can simply make more of the Turbo-charge Smoothie, put it into a flask and have it for lunch.

▲ The Juice Master's Turbo Salad – Light Version (page 213)

▲ Green Veggie Power Soup (page 219) – Best to make it the night before, heat it in the morning and put it in a flask ready for lunch. The recipe makes enough for four so you'll have some for another day or so.

▲ The Juice Master's Turbo Power Sandwich (page 224)

▲ The Juice Master's Protein Snack Attack (page 229) – You may have as much of this lunch as you like.

▲ 1 tub Rachel's Organic Live Yogurt with Honey (available in supermarkets) – You may add some berries or fresh mango if you wish.

Late Afternoon/Early Evening

▪ Time for your second main workout of the day.

▪ Choose from the following menu:

Dinner Options

▲ The Juice Master's Turbo Salad – Main Course Version (page 214)

▲ Green Veggie Power Soup (page 219)

▲ The Juice Master's Green Power Smoothie (page 196)

▲ Jasey's Fish Kebabs with Pineapple and Steamed Veggies (page 236)

▲ Honey-glazed Vegetables (page 235)

▲ The Juice Master's Fish 'n' Chips (page 238)

▲ Salsa Salmon (page 244)

▲ Oven-steamed Chicken and Vegetables (page 234)

▲ Thyme for Tuna (page 233)

▲ Alternatively, you are free to use any of your own recipes that consist of a protein-based meal (fish/chicken/tofu/Quorn) with plenty of salad and/or stir-fried veggies. This combination gives you an immense choice.

▨ Do a 10-minute visualization of your goals while breathing deeply and listening to relaxing music.

▨ Do not eat anything else before you sleep but keep drinking plenty of water, herbal teas or hot water with lemon or lime.

▨ Prepare your workout clothes and get to bed – you want to be up early tomorrow!

Days 8 to 12 (Monday to Friday)

Days 8 to 12 are very similar to days 1 to 5. Always remember you are welcome to make your own lunch and dinner as long as you stick to the rules of the programme.

Morning

- Get up in plenty of time for your morning workout and to make juice.
- Drink a glass of water before you do anything else, preferably warm water with lemon or lime.
- Spend a good few minutes breathing deeply, asking your three questions and doing your visualization. Once again, please make sure you don't skip this part of the programme.
- Put on your gym/walking clothes and head to the park/gym or wherever you are choosing to do your morning physical wake-up.
- Put music on and begin your morning workout of 45–60 minutes.
- Make a Turbo-charge Smoothie (page 195) and drink slowly. If you are not hungry, put it in a flask and have it mid-morning.

NOTE: If you are waking up and going straight to the gym, make your smoothie before you go, seal it in a flask and ask the people at the gym to leave it in their fridge. You can then drink it in the sauna or when you come out.

Lunch

- Get some oxygen circulating as often as possible by doing some deep-breathing exercises. Also do some visualization, as the more your brain sees the direction it wants to go in, the more likely it is to get there. If you have time, do some sort of very light exercise.
- Choose any of The Juice Master's Turbo Lunches below:

Lunch Options

- ▲ The Juice Master's Turbo Salad – Light Version (page 213)
- ▲ Watercress and Baby Leek Soup (page 221)
- ▲ Green Veggie Power Soup (page 219) – Best to make it the night before, heat it in the morning and put it in a flask ready for lunch. The recipe makes enough for four so you'll have some for another day or so.
- ▲ The Juice Master's Green Power Smoothie (page 196) – Again, this can be made in advance when you are making your morning Turbo-charge Smoothie. If you prefer, you can simply make more of the Turbo-charge Smoothie, put it into a flask and have it for lunch.
- ▲ The Juice Master's Turbo-power Sandwich (page 224)
- ▲ The Juice Master's Protein Snack Attack (page 229)
- ▲ 1 whole tub Rachel's Organic Live Yogurt with Honey (available from supermarkets)
- ▲ Jasey's Veggie Sushi Rolls (page 226)

After Work – Late Afternoon/Early Evening

- Time for your second main workout of the day. You can choose to eat at this point and work out later in evening, if that suits you better. The reason I have chosen after work is because it fits in with most people's schedules and is the time when most people look for food and the sofa – where they often stay all night!
- Choose from the following menu:

Dinner Options

▲ The Juice Master's Turbo Salad – Main Course Version (page 214)

▲ Green Veggie Power Soup (page 219)

▲ The Juice Master's Green Power Smoothie (page 196)

▲ Salmon with Vegetable Courgette (page 242)

▲ Juicy Stir-fried Monkfish 'n' Veggie Special (page 239)

▲ Jasey's Fish Kebabs with Pineapple and Steamed Vegetables (page 236)

▲ Honey-glazed Vegetables (page 235)

▲ Thyme for Tuna (page 233)

▲ Alternatively, you are free to use any of your own recipes that consist of a protein-based meal (fish/chicken/tofu/Quorn) with plenty of salad and/or stir-fried veggies. This combination gives you an immense choice.

■ Do a 10-minute visualization of your goals while breathing deeply and listening to relaxing music.

■ Do not eat anything else before you sleep but keep drinking plenty of water, herbal teas or hot water with lemon or lime.

■ Get prepared for tomorrow and go to bed as you want to be up early.

Day 13 (Saturday)

Morning

- Get up in plenty of time for morning workout and to make a Turbo-charge Smoothie.
- Drink a glass of water before you do anything else, preferably warm water with lemon or lime.
- Spend a few minutes breathing deeply, asking your three questions and doing your visualization. **THIS IS STILL IMPORTANT!**
- Put on your gym/walking clothes and head to the park/gym or wherever you are choosing to do your morning physical wake-up.
- Put music on and begin your morning workout of 45–60 minutes.
- Make a Turbo-charge Smoothie or a Turbo-charge Weekend Breakfast Smoothie (pages 195 and 200).

Lunch

- As it's the weekend, chances are you'll have more time during the day to get your body moving! Remember, you are looking to create a new pattern of behaviour over the 14 days and to move your body as much as possible. Once again, this doesn't mean battering yourself; it just means taking time to go for a long walk, do some deep breathing or, if you are reasonably healthy, increasing your exercise at weekends.
- Prepare/have lunch from the following menus choices:

  ▲ The Juice Master's Green Power Smoothie (page 196) – Again, this can be made in advance when you are making your morning Turbo-charge Smoothie. If you prefer, you can simply make more of the Turbo-charge Smoothie, put it into a flask and have it for lunch.
  ▲ The Juice Master's Turbo Salad – Light Version (page 213)
  ▲ Green Veggie Power Soup (page 219) – Best to make it the night before, heat it in the morning and put it in a flask ready for

lunch. The recipe makes enough for four so you'll have some for another day or so.

▲ The Juice Master's Turbo-power Sandwich (page 224)

▲ The Juice Master's Protein Snack Attack (page 229) – You may have as much as you like.

▲ 1 tub Rachel's Organic Live Yogurt with Honey (available in supermarkets) – You may add some berries or fresh mango.

Late Afternoon/Early Evening

■ Time for your second main workout of the day.

■ Choose from the following menu:

Dinner Options

▲ The Juice Master's Turbo Salad – Main Course Version (page 214)

▲ Green Veggie Power Soup (page 219)

▲ The Juice Master's Green Power Smoothie (page 196)

▲ Jasey's Fish Kebabs with Pineapple and Steamed Veggies (page 236)

▲ Honey-glazed Vegetables (page 235)

▲ Salsa Salmon (page 244)

▲ Oven-steamed Chicken and Vegetables (page 234)

▲ Thyme for Tuna (page 233)

▲ Alternatively, you are free to use any of your own recipes that consist of a protein-based meal (fish/chicken/tofu/Quorn) with plenty of salad and/or stir-fried veggies. This combination gives you an immense choice.

■ Do a 10-minute visualization of your goals while breathing deeply and listening to relaxing music.

■ Do not eat anything else before you sleep but keep drinking plenty of water, herbal teas or hot water with lemon or lime.

■ No need to set the alarm as it's Sunday tomorrow and you get to have a lie-in!

Day 14 (Sunday)

The End of the Programme – The Start of a New Lease of Life

Firstly – CONGRATULATIONS! You have made it this far. This means you are one of the rare people who have not only read the book but also acted on the information in it. Although this is the final day of the Turbo-charge Your Life programme, I sincerely hope it's not the final day of doing whatever it takes to bring your life to the next level.

Two weeks of watching very little TV, reading some inspiring books, getting lots of exercise, visualizing your goals, feeling grateful each day and consuming the right food and drinks should have made a significant difference to how you look and feel. I genuinely hope you decide to make it a lifestyle choice. See 'Keeping it Real *After* the Programme' (page 187) for advice on adapting the programme to fit in with you and *your* new lifestyle.

However, before we get into that, we still have the last day of the 'set' programme to complete. To make sure you get the most out of it, every meal is 100 per cent natural, and it's the only day I will ask you to stick fully to the menu provided.

- Wake up at your leisure – it's Sunday after all.
- Have your glass of hot water with lemon/lime.
- Go for a one-hour workout.
- Shower/change.
- Make a Turbo-charge Smoothie and drink slowly.
- Read the Sunday papers.

Lunch

■ Just three choices here:

Lunch Options

▲ The Juice Master's Turbo Salad – Light Version (page 213)

▲ Green Veggie Power Soup (page 219)

▲ The Juice Master's Green Power Smoothie (page 196)

Late Afternoon/Early Evening

■ Time for your second main workout of the day.

■ Choose from this little lot:

Dinner Options

▲ The Juice Master's Turbo Salad – Main Course Version (page 214)

▲ Green Veggie Power Soup (page 219)

▲ The Juice Master's Green Power Smoothie (page 196)

Keeping it Real *After* the Programme

Keeping it real is essential to *lifelong* success. This means accepting we are all human and have our weak moments from time to time – yes, that includes me! Being real means understanding that none of us is perfect, and that we'll never truly achieve our goals if we try playing the 'perfection game' on a daily basis.

It's What You Do *Most* of the Time that Determines Your Health

In an ideal world, we'd never have anything with refined sugar in it. We'd never drink alcohol, caffeine or anything containing artificial chemicals. We'd consume nothing but fruit, vegetables, whole grains, lean proteins and freshly extracted juices, and we would exercise twice a day, every day, for ever more. This, as most of you will know, doesn't happen in the real world. We will always have the *odd* dietary and exercise indiscretion, and as long as we don't let it spiral out of proportion, there's actually not a lot wrong with it. On a physical level, the body can easily deal with pretty much anything from time to time; we have to make sure that we are just as resilient mentally.

For some people, certain foods and drinks are like nicotine: they can trigger an almost instant reversal of dietary behaviour. When someone has been without cigarettes for weeks, months or even years, just one puff can trigger the old pattern of behaviour, and they can be back on a packet a day before they know it. The same principle applies to food or, to be more accurate, drug-like foods and drinks. Even a slight indiscretion can lead some people back to all their old eating habits. If you are aware that you are one of these people then be very careful if you ever have a dietary indiscretion. There's no need for it to spiral out of control as long as you are aware of what's happening and you 'clean up' the next day.

The general rule is not to have days and days of indiscretions, otherwise the old foods and behaviours take refuge before you know it, and you'll find it very tricky to 'kick-start' yourself again. Once you've made the change and completed the 14-day programme, your new behaviour pattern should have developed sufficiently for your brain to want to keep it.

Airport Day

If you ever see me at an airport or on an aeroplane you can almost bet your bottom dollar that I won't be eating just salad and having juice. Chances are I'll be tucking into some sort of sandwich, and sometimes even eating the absolute rubbish they serve on the plane. Why? Well, airports are one of the few places where it is genuinely hard to find some decent, natural food, and finding a juice bar is almost impossible (unless you're in Stansted Airport where you have Love Juice – yes, that's the name!).

Having said that, this could easily be seen as a 'but' excuse. If I really wanted to I could prepare some decent food for the flight and bring a packed lunch. However, as the *vast majority* of the time I live an extremely healthy lifestyle, and given that I'm no longer overweight, I know I don't have to be 'anal' about such days and can grab whatever food is available. Often, though, I will actually choose to bring some fruit on a plane, and I always make sure I drink plenty of water because of the dehydrating effect of flying. But if I forget to prepare I will eat whatever is there … to some degree. Well, come on – even I can't eat everything on those plastic 'food' trays; half of it is 'mystery food'.

Now, clearly, if your job involves having to commute by plane every day or once or twice a week, then airport day doesn't apply to you. You will need to look at ways to eat healthily on such days; such as taking fruit and/or a packed lunch.

I have called it airport day but it could just as well be 'theme park day' or 'staying at a hotel day' – it's a day when it's difficult to get decent food and so you choose the best of what's available or prepare and bring your own. If you have an airport day scheduled during the 14-day programme then you must make certain you prepare: there are to be *no* exceptions whatsoever during this time.

Flexibility is important. You must allow for the occasional airport day and not drive yourself cuckoo. Once again, though, even on airport day, you must avoid foods or drinks which can trigger old patterns of behaviour. For example, I would never, ever have a cigarette again – even on airport day. This is because I don't want to, and it could cause a knock-on reaction and lead me back into the smoking trap. For many people, just a sniff of wheat, white sugar or chocolate is enough to get them back into old ways.

Give the Body More Credit

However, if you know that certain 'rubbish' foods will *not* trigger an emotional hook, then it is imperative that you feel free to have them from time to time. The human body will do its utmost to make sure it turns whatever comes in into usable fuel.

The body can put up with eating rubbish for many years, but eventually it takes its toll. It will start to break down, and disease in one form or another (like weight gain) will set in. It is therefore essential that the *majority* of what comes into the body is in the form of 'live', natural, easy-to-digest, nutritionally rich food and drink. You are still most welcome to have the *odd* exception from time to time, but you must never make the exception the rule. The danger is that airport day becomes every day, and before you know where you are, you're back in the thick of it. Mental freedom and a non-diet mentality are the keys to lifelong success.

Ten Simple Rules for Permanent, Healthy Weight Loss

On a physical level, losing weight and keeping it off really couldn't be easier. If you adopt my 10 simple rules and make sure you rarely digress, you will not only lose weight but, much more importantly, you will keep it off and you will be healthy.

1. **CHEW YOUR FOOD THOROUGHLY – *Your stomach doesn't have teeth!***

   The enzymes in your saliva are more efficient at breaking down your food than those found in your stomach. By eating slowly as opposed to 'wafting it down' you will actually get to taste your food (often a novel concept), improve your digestion and, because you are giving time for your body to acknowledge that it has been fed, you feel fuller quicker and so eat less!

2. **EAT ONLY WHEN GENUINLY PHYSICALLY HUNGRY – *You cannot feed an emotion with food!***

   Often when we think we want food we actually want to change the way we feel. However, it is worth remembering before you think 'food' can cheer you up that not only can you never satisfy an emotional void with food, but anything you eat when you are not genuinely physically hungry gets stored in the body as FAT! The real pleasure in eating is in the ending of a genuine hunger; if you aren't hungry you won't get any genuine pleasure from eating.

3. **STOP EATING WHEN YOU ARE *JUST* FULL – *This is one of the key elements to permanent weight loss.***

   If you try to fill a 8 oz glass with 10 ounces of liquid, you will obviously get an overspill. The same principle applies with food, even if it's healthy food. Eat more than your body wants and you will get an overspill, only you can't just mop up this overspill as it will be around your waist, hips and thighs in the form of FAT!

4. **EXERCISE FOR 30–60 MINUTES TWICE A DAY –** *Your body was designed to move!*

   Walk, run, hop, skip, bounce, swim, ski, snowboard, do some weights – anything – but just get that body moving – really moving! Exercise helps to clean the body of dead cells, clears the mind, reduces stress and speeds up your basal metabolic rate, helping to burn fuel efficiently.

5. **DRINK 2 LITRES OF WATER A DAY –** *Hydration is key!*

   Often when we think we are hungry it's the body crying out for water. This is why before you even think of food you should have a glass of water to make sure you weren't just thirsty.

6. **EAT NO 'MAN-MADE' CARBOHYDRATES AFTER 6PM** *(no potatoes, pasta or bread) with the exception of wild/brown rice.*

   This doesn't mean all the time – remember 'Keeping it Real *After* the Programme' – but this is one of the best physical tools to drop the excess pounds and keep them off. Sometimes you don't even need to know why something works, just that it does – and this works!

7. **60–70% OF YOUR DIET SHOULD CONSIST OF WATER-RICH 'LIVE' FOODS –** *The body needs the right fuel*

   You can 'thin' by simply eating less, no matter what food it is, but if you want to be slim and healthy the majority of what you eat should consist of fresh fruits and vegetables. They are virtually pre-digested by the plant, are high in water content and furnish the body with the right fuel for optimum health.

8. **GET JUICED!** *If you can't eat it, drink it!*

   The easiest way to get good quality 'live' nutrition in your system is to have it in liquid form, and the easiest way to do that is to juice some fresh fruits and vegetables. A glass of freshly extracted juice a day is one of the best health insurances you can invest in.

9. **DO NOT EAT ANY PROCESSED FOOD FOR THREE HOURS BEFORE YOU SLEEP**

   When you sleep your metabolic rate slows down and efficient digestion becomes harder. This is also why many people don't feel hungry in the morning, skip breakfast and often feel groggy.

10. **DO SOME WEIGHT-RESISTING EXERCISE EVERY OTHER DAY**

    This helps to tone muscles which in turn helps to burn fat while you sleep!

The Juice Master's 10 Commandments

1. Be grateful for what you do have, not what you think you can't have.
2. Visualize your goals on a daily basis.
3. Feed your body nourishing foods.
4. Feed your mind nourishing information.
5. Have a glass of freshly extracted juice daily.
6. Treat others as you would like others to treat you.
7. Take physical exercise and get plenty of fresh air every day.
8. Do something worthwhile for someone else every day.
9. Tell the people close to you that you love them.
10. Understand at any given moment you have the choice – either get busy living or get busy dying!

recipes RECIPES recipes

recipes recipes recipes recipes recipes recipes recipes recipes recipes

recipes recipes recipes recipes recipes recipes recipes

recipes recipes recipes recipes RECIPES recipes

recipes recipes RECIPES recipes recipes

recipes recipes recipes RECIPES recipes

recipes recipes recipes recipes recipes recipes

recipes recipes recipes recipes recipes recipes recipes recipes recipes recipes recipes

RECIPES

recipes recipes recipes recipes recipes recipes

recipes recipes recipes recipes

recipes recipes recipes recipes

recipes recipes RECIPES recipes recipes RECIPES

recipes recipes recipes recipes recipes recipes recipes

RECIPES recipes recipes recipes recipes RECIPES recipes recipes recipes recipes

recipes RECIPES recipes

Juices&
Power Smoothies*

Pure liquid gold – there is no better way to describe what you are getting when you consume freshly extracted juices and freshly made smoothies. Each mouthful provides your system with easy-to-digest 'live' nutrients, which not only feed every cell in the body, but also replenish your life bank accounts. Quite simply, they are the best health-insurance policy you'll ever invest in.

You cannot possibly get the same taste or benefits from shop-bought juices and smoothies. The only way to get the incredible benefits of 'live' juice is to make it yourself. So pull out your juicer and blender and GET JUICING!

*Wherever possible use organic produce. However, if you can't get your hands on any, non-organic is fine but remember to wash it thoroughly before use.

The Juice Master's
Turbo-charge Smoothie

Serves 1

This smoothie features heavily in the Turbo-charge Your Life programme, and for good reason. Not only is it rich and incredibly creamy but it's also loaded with all six essential dietary needs. The blended avocado provides fibre and plenty of satisfying 'good' fat and protein. Packed with vitamins, minerals and antioxidants, this smoothie has been designed to nourish every cell in your body.

¼ cucumber
1 stick celery
½ small pineapple, peeled and chopped
Handful of spinach leaves
¼ lime, peeled
4 Golden Delicious apples, chopped
Flesh of ½ ripe avocado
Small handful of ice

Juice the cucumber, celery, pineapple, spinach, lime and 3½ apples. Place the avocado and the remaining ½ apple in a blender, together with the juice mixture and ice. Give a good whiz for 45 seconds. Pour into a glass and enjoy!

A *truly* **amazing meal** in a GLASS.

The Juice Master's
Green Power Smoothie

Serves 1–2

Although similar to the Turbo-charge Smoothie, the addition of ginger, lemon, different apples and more celery makes a subtle change. Again, this is a meal in a glass, so take your time with it and drink only enough to make you full – don't think the more you drink the better because that's not how the body works.

2 sticks celery
½ small cucumber
3 Royal Gala apples
1 inch fresh ginger
2 cups spinach
½ small pineapple, peeled
½ lemon, peeled
Flesh of 1 ripe avocado
Small handful of ice

Juice everything apart from the avocado and ice. Pour the juice into a blender along with the ice and avocado and give a good whiz. Pour into a glass and enjoy!

The Juice Master's
Ultimate Smoothie

Serves 2

This really is the ultimate. Rich in beta-carotene, potassium, calcium, iron, zinc, chlorophyll, essential fats, good proteins and excellent carbohydrates, it's also brimming with antioxidants. If making for one simply halve all ingredients.

4 Golden Delicious apples
2 sticks celery
4 carrots
1 cup spinach
1 cup broccoli
½ yellow pepper
½ orange pepper
¼ lime, peeled
Flesh of 1 ripe avocado
Handful of ice

Juice 3 of the apples, the celery, carrots, spinach, broccoli, peppers and lime. Place the avocado in a blender together with the juice and add the ice. Whiz for 1 minute, pour into a glass and enjoy!

Although **VERY FILLING,** it's *incredibly* easy for the body to digest.

The Juice Master's
Mean, Green Wake-up Machine

Serves 1–2

This amazing juice will certainly give you a bit of a zing in the morning. The smell of freshly extracted ginger and lime juice alone is enough to wake you up. Loaded with vitamins and minerals, the juice will also bring life to every cell in your body.

Drink just one of these a day and you will get more live nutrients than most people consume in a week!

½ **cucumber**
1 **stick celery**
1 **cup spinach**
6 **green apples (preferably Golden Delicious)**
¼ **lime, peeled**
½ **inch fresh ginger**

Simply juice all the ingredients, pour into a glass over ice, drink and enjoy!

This **juice** is as *good for you* as it is **refreshing.**

Green Means Go

Serves 2

Get up and go in this case. I'm sure the thought of having green vegetables for breakfast is quite alien for many of you. However, this juice is beautifully sweet and packed with power. It's a great choice for when you want to get out there and show them what you are made of!

The combination of pineapple and apple makes it a fantastic system cleanser as well as packing it with vitamin C, dietary fibre, folic acid and beta-carotene. The spinach gives a small amount of viscous juice, but you don't need much of this mineral-packed vegetable. Spinach also contains more protein than most other vegetables. The ginger root is a great aid to digestion and will help settle any nauseous feelings in the morning. The lime gives this juice a great kick as well as providing it with folic acid, beta-carotene, vitamin C and calcium.

1 small pineapple, topped, tailed and peeled
2 apples of your choice
4 good handfuls of spinach
1 inch root ginger
2 inches fennel
¼ lime
Handful of ice

Cut the pineapple and apples into feeder chute-size pieces and juice. A handy tip (depending on your juicer) is to bunch the spinach up really tightly in the feeder and follow it by feeding through something hard like the apples – it just makes juicing a little easier on the machine. Put the ginger, fennel and lime through midway as well to make sure you get all the juice from them. Once all juiced, pour into a tall glass over the ice and get going!

The Juice Master's
Turbo-charge Weekend Breakfast Smoothie

Serves 1–2

This smoothie is packed with age-defying and disease-preventing antioxidants. It's a great breakfast smoothie, giving a good shot of vitamin C, and has a lovely crunchy consistency – good to get your teeth into! It's also a welcome change on days 6, 7 and 13 of the Turbo-charge Your Life programme.

1 small pineapple, peeled
2 handfuls of blueberries (or any berries you can get, fresh or frozen)
4 tbsp live yoghurt
Handful of soaked almonds (best to soak overnight but not essential)
1 tbsp organic Manuka honey

Juice the pineapple and 1 handful of the blueberries. Pour into a blender and whiz with the yoghurt, remaining blueberries, nuts and honey until smooth. Pour into a glass and enjoy this beautiful and filling smoothie for breakfast.

Salad **in a Glass**

Serves 1

An alternative to the traditional salad on a plate. Tomatoes are rich in lycopene, which is important in helping to prevent heart disease and cancer. This juice is also full of potassium, folic acid, vitamin C, beta-carotene and calcium – a fantastic cleanser.

1 stick celery
2 tomatoes
¼ cucumber
Handful of salad leaves of your choice
2 carrots, topped and tailed
1 apple (preferably Golden Delicious)
Handful of ice

Juice everything and add ice.

Nerve Calmer

Serves 1

If your day ahead involves an interview, exam, big meeting with your boss or any-thing that makes your stomach somersault, then this juice really is a winner. Ginger and fennel are a soothing combination. The fennel gives this juice a lovely aniseed/liquorice taste but is incredibly potent, so add slowly until you are happy with the taste. The apples provide a touch of sweetness along with dietary fibre. This juice is also high in vitamin C, potassium and calcium.

½ fennel, outer part removed
2 apples, cut into feeder chute-size pieces
½ inch root ginger
Handful of ice

Juice all the ingredients and pour into a glass over ice.

The Juice Master's
Fruit Salad

Serves 1

No, not the halfpenny chews we loved as kids, but a beautiful juice you will want to make again and again. Packed with vitamins C and E, beta-carotene, antioxidants, calcium, phosphorous, potassium and folic acid, this juice is a fantastic digestive and system cleanser, and is also great for your skin.

1 orange
1 apple
1 kiwi
Handful of grapes
Handful of strawberries
Handful of ice

Peel the orange with a knife, leaving as much of the pith on as possible. Cut the orange, apple and kiwi into feeder chute-size pieces. Juice everything and pour into a glass over ice. Savour and enjoy!

It will pick you up and give you boundless energy.

Cranberry **Delight**

Serves 1

This juice has an incredibly crisp taste and a plethora of nutrients including beta-carotene, folic acid, vitamin C, calcium, chlorine, magnesium, phosphorous and potassium. It is also high in antioxidants and great for the digestion and urinary tract.

1 mango
1 orange
125g (4½oz) cranberries
1 tsp Manuka honey
½ inch root ginger
Handful of ice

Peel the mango, remove the stone and chop into feeder chute-size pieces. Peel the orange with a knife, leaving as much of the white pith on as possible, and juice these along with the ginger and cranberries (you can leave a couple of cranberries for decoration if you wish). Pour the juice into a blender with the honey and ginger and give a quick whiz. Transfer to a long glass and decorate with the remaining cranberries if you wish.

The Juice Master's
Energy Boost

Serves 1–2

For that simple injection of energy that is so often needed mid-afternoon, try reaching for this natural smoothie rather than for a chocolate bar.

This smoothie will boost your energy naturally and satisfy any hunger pangs that may be starting to surface. It is also excellent if you are working out and looking to gain some muscle mass.

1 mango
½ medium pineapple
2 dates
1 banana
3 tbsp live plain yoghurt
1 tsp desiccated coconut
½ tsp organic Manuka honey
Handful of ice

Peel the mango and cut the flesh around the stone. Peel the pineapple and juice along with the mango. Remove the stones from the dates. Pour the mango and pineapple juice into a blender along with all the remaining ingredients. Give a good whiz, pour into a glass and enjoy.

For **best results,** drink *half an hour* after your **workout.**

Midday Melon Juice

Serves 1–2

This juice has a real 'wow factor' because of its amazing colour and taste. It's packed with beta-carotene, vitamin C, phyto-chemicals, folic acid, calcium, magnesium, phosphorous and potassium.

Melon juice is also incredibly beneficial to drink on its own due to its high water content.

½ small watermelon
2 pomegranates
¼ lemon, peeled
100g (4oz) raspberries
Handful of ice

Scoop out the flesh of the watermelon and remove the pomegranate seeds, reserving a few for decoration if you wish.

Juice the melon flesh, lemon and the rest of the pomegranate seeds with the raspberries.

Serve over the ice and decorate with the reserved pomegranate seeds – you will have everyone 'ooohhhhing' with this delicious, delightful-looking juice.

The Juice Master's
Breath of Fresh Air

Serves 1

If your breath is feeling and tasting a little less than fresh after lunch, this beautiful juice will not only lift you physically and mentally, but will also leave your breath as fresh as the morning dew!

Bad breath can be caused by poor digestion, constipation, illness, lack of food, dental decay, gum disease, coffee, tobacco and too much rich or spicy food.

2 carrots
1 apple
55g (2oz) parsley
Handful of ice

Top and tail the carrots and chop the apple and carrots into feeder chute-size pieces. Juice everything and pour over the ice. Drink and feel your senses coming alive.

CARROTS and PARSLEY are **especially good** for freshening **breath.**

The Juice Master's
Morning Reviver

Serves 1

This juice has a fantastically cool taste so is particularly good for a warm, sunny morning. The grapefruit makes it a great cleanser as well as packing it with vitamin C. Mint provides a distinctive flavour, helps digestion and leaves a fresh taste in your mouth – I'm sure this can often be a huge welcome, particularly for your partner!

1 grapefruit, peeled
½ pineapple
6 mint leaves
Handful of ice

Juice the grapefruit and pineapple and transfer to a blender with the mint leaves and ice. Give a good whiz, pour and enjoy. If this one doesn't make you raise an eyebrow, I don't know what will!

The Juice Master's
Sunrise

Serves 1

Whether the morning sky is a lovely pink hue or whether clouds are blocking all hope of sunlight, this juice will emanate not only the colour but also the sunny feeling that is so often needed first thing.

This juice is brimming with vitamins C and E, beta-carotene, calcium, potassium, folic acid and antioxidants. It's a great liver and kidney cleanser and a good energy enhancer. The sprinkle of wheat germ adds a boost of vitamins B and E and fibre.

1 orange, peeled
Handful of strawberries
3 carrots, topped and tailed
1 lemon, peeled
Sprinkle of wheat germ
Handful of ice

Juice together the orange, strawberries, carrots and lemon. Once juiced, stir in the wheat germ and pour into a glass over ice. A beautiful array of sunshine colours to tantalize your taste buds!

Power
Salads

'Rabbit food!' That's the most common reaction when people think of salads. No doubt this is largely due to what passes for salads in most restaurants. You know, a few bits of iceberg lettuce, a couple of ropey-looking tomato slices and cucumber. No wonder 'salads' don't seem to entice.

Before I got into this healthy food lark I would never have thought you could be satisfied by eating just a salad. However, not only do the following salads taste wonderful, they are also incredibly filling. Because they are full of water-rich 'live' nutrients, you can have as much or as little as you like.

They have got to be the quickest and easiest meals to prepare, and they look and taste great. You can indulge as a main meal or serve as a side salad – just increase or decrease the quantities. They can also be kept in the fridge and used for sandwiches or for filling a warm wholemeal pitta.

So open your mind and try some of these power-packed salads.

Green Salad **with Mustard Dressing**

Serves 1

The spinach, rocket, watercress and alfalfa sprouts alone contain vitamins B, E, C and K, choline, folic acid, beta-carotene, sulphur, iron, calcium, silicon, zinc, potassium, magnesium and iodine. The ingredients in this salad benefit the respiratory tract and lungs; support kidney and liver function; improve vision; and help arthritis and gout. In just one salad we have an easy-to-digest combination of natural proteins, carbohydrates and essential fatty acids. One thing you cannot say is that it's 'just a salad' – enjoy!

Handful of baby spinach leaves
Handful of watercress
Small handful of rocket
Handful of alfalfa sprouts
2 spring onions, chopped
½ red onion, peeled and sliced
Small handful coriander leaves
7 baby tomatoes
2 tablespoons cold-pressed virgin olive oil

THE DRESSING

4 tbsp olive oil
Juice of 1 lemon
1 tbsp mustard powder
1 clove garlic, peeled and chopped

This is so simple it surely can't be right! You basically throw all the greens, onions and tomatoes into a bowl and toss really well.

To make the dressing, mix together the oil, lemon juice, mustard powder and garlic and drizzle it creatively over the salad. So simple yet so tasty!

Brown Rice Salad

Serves 2

This is incredibly simple to make, tastes delicious, is incredibly good for you and, unlike carbohydrates such as pasta and bread, you will still feel light, yet satisfied, after eating it.

The rice is full of vitamins and minerals, and is an excellent source of fibre, designed to keep you on the move! The garlic and onions are a natural antibiotic; they also help to prevent blood clots and will keep colds at bay. The olive oil contains essential fatty acids, excellent for the skin, and the dried dates are an excellent source of natural carbohydrate. All in all, it's one hell of an amazing salad.

100g (4oz) long-grain brown rice or wild rice
2 tbsp (30ml) cold-pressed virgin olive oil
1 tbsp (15ml) cider vinegar
½ clove garlic, crushed
½ tbsp fresh thyme, finely chopped
35g (1½oz) organic cheese, grated
4 spring onions, finely chopped
1 stick of celery, thinly sliced
2 dried dates, chopped
Sea salt
Freshly ground black pepper

Cook the rice in a large pan of salted, boiling water (for full cooking instructions please refer to the packet). Rinse, drain and cool the rice.

Meanwhile, mix together thoroughly the oil, vinegar, garlic and thyme to make a dressing.

Place all the ingredients in a large bowl, add the rice and oil dressing and mix thoroughly.

Leave to stand for 30 minutes before serving.

The Juice Master's
Turbo Salad

Light Version

Serves 1 peckish person

**1 cup mixed spinach and
    rocket leaves**

½ cup watercress

⅛ cup red cabbage, grated

¼ carrot, grated

¼ small cucumber, diced

¼ cup broccoli, grated

**½ sweet pepper (any colour),
    diced finely**

4 black or green olives

Egg cupful of cold-pressed olive oil

Balsamic vinegar

1 lemon

1 lime

**Flesh of 1 large avocado,
    diced into large chunks**

Why it's Sooooo Good!

This salad is amazing on both a taste and health front. It contains the six dietary needs in abundance, including 'good fats' in the form of avocados, olives and cold-pressed olive oil. Just about every ingredient contains amino acids (the building blocks for protein) and natural carbohydrates. On top of that it has an array of bio-available vitamins and minerals, including beta-carotene, calcium, iron, potassium, vitamin C, folic acid and chlorophyll – the life blood of the plant – providing your cells with life-giving oxygen.

Place the spinach, rocket and watercress leaves on a plate or in a small salad bowl. Top with the red cabbage, carrot, cucumber, broccoli, pepper and olives. Add olive oil and balsamic vinegar and juice from half the lemon and lime. Toss together. Place the avocado chunks on top and squeeze over the juice from the remaining lemon and lime.

Hot Tip!
Feel free to cook up some white meat, fish, tofu or Quorn to mix in.

The Juice Master's
Turbo Salad

Main Course Version

Serves 1 hungry person

1 cup spinach leaves

1 cup rocket leaves

½ cup watercress

⅛ cup red cabbage, grated

½ carrot, grated

¼ small cucumber, diced

¼ cup broccoli grated

½ sweet pepper (any colour),
   diced

4 black or green olives

Egg cupful of cold-pressed olive oil

Balsamic vinegar

1 lemon

1 lime

Flesh of 1 large avocado,
   diced into large chunks

Why it's Sooooo Good!

For all the same reasons as The Juice Master's Turbo Salad – Light Version, just this time you get even more! This salad is rich in silica, helping the hair, nails and skin. The cabbage is superb for many digestive and intestinal problems, such as bowel infections, parasites and colitis, and the broccoli is one of Nature's true super-foods, helpful for high blood pressure, liver problems and constipation. The grated carrot helps to reduce inflammation of the mucous membranes in the intestines and respiratory tract. This really is one hell of a power salad!

Place the spinach, rocket and watercress leaves on a plate or in a small salad bowl. Top with the red cabbage, carrot, cucumber, broccoli, pepper and olives. Add olive oil and balsamic vinegar and juice from half the lemon and lime. Toss together. Place the avocado chunks on top and squeeze over the juice from the remaining lemon and lime.

Avocado **and Tofu Salad**

Serves 1

If you think eating tofu is one short step from the funny farm, please feel free to replace it with some fish or chicken. However, tofu is a very good source of protein and, once mixed with the other ingredients, it adds a nice texture. This power salad is packed with so many vitamins, minerals, essential fatty acids, natural carbohydrates and good proteins that there just isn't enough space to list them all.

2 handfuls of mixed green leaves
   (spinach, rocket, watercress, lettuce)
100g (4oz) cubed tofu
55g (2oz) cherry tomatoes
30g (1oz) alfalfa sprouts
2 tbsp pitted olives (green or black)
½ avocado

THE DRESSING
½ clove garlic
Pinch of dried chilli
3 tbsp lemon juice
1 tbsp olive oil
55g (2oz) almonds

Put the mixed green leaves, tofu, tomatoes, alfalfa sprouts and pitted olives into a serving dish. Scoop out and add the avocado flesh.

Crush the garlic and put in a bowl or screw-top jar along with the dried chilli, lemon juice and olive oil. Give it a good mix or shake and pour over the salad. Give the salad a good toss so the ingredients are covered with the oil. Finally, crush the almonds so they are ground into little bits – you can do this by putting them in a little plastic bag and crushing with a rolling pin. Sprinkle the nuts over the salad and enjoy.

Grilled Vegetable Salad

Serves 1

This salad is a blaze of beautiful colours and tastes to match. It can be made in minutes and is fantastic when you have friends round. As with all of the power salads, it's rich in vitamins and minerals, easy to digest, and you can have as much as you like until you are full!

1 red pepper

3 asparagus tips

½ small courgette, sliced

Handful of rocket

Handful of watercress

2 small spring onions

2 fresh red chillies, deseeded and finely
   chopped

Good handful of mixed fresh herbs
   (coriander, basil, mint, flat-leaf parsley),
   torn roughly into pieces

THE DRESSING

2 tbsp lemon juice

5 tbsp olive oil

Freshly ground black pepper

Blacken the pepper by placing it under the grill, turning until all sides are black. Wrap in clingfilm or put in a sandwich or freezer bag for 5 minutes until cool. This method steams the skin of the pepper, making peeling and deseeding easier. Remove the skin and seeds and chop it up.

In a very hot ridged pan, lightly char the asparagus and courgette on both sides.

Throw everything except the asparagus into a bowl and mix well. Place the asparagus on top. Make the dressing by putting the lemon juice and olive oil into a screw-top jar and shaking really well. Pour over the salad and season with black pepper.

Souper
Stuff

The next best thing to juice, soup is ideal for getting loads of fresh vegetables into your system in a way that's extremely easy to digest. Unlike juice, soup still contains a lot of fibre.

On a cold winter's day, few things can beat the taste and texture of a well-made, freshly prepared soup.

The following soup recipes – my personal top five – are all brimming with vitamins, minerals, antioxidants and taste.

Squash **Soup**

Serves 1–2

This soup is packed full of potassium, vitamins A and C, folic acid, loads of anti-oxidants and even some good bacteria. It's easy to make and, like all of these soups, easy on the digestive system.

500ml (16fl oz) vegetable stock
750g (1lb 10 oz) squash, cut into cubes
2 red onions, chopped
2 garlic cloves, halved
60ml (2fl oz) live yoghurt
¼ tsp ground nutmeg

Put the stock and 500ml (15fl oz) of water into a heavy-based pan and bring to the boil. Add the squash, onions and garlic and return to the boil. Reduce the heat slightly and cook for 15 minutes or until the squash is smooth.

Drain the vegetables in a colander, reserving the liquid. Purée the squash mixture until smooth, either in a blender or with a hand masher (you may need to add some of the reserved liquid to make mashing a little easier). Return the squash purée to the pan and stir in enough reserved liquid to reach the preferred consistency. Season to taste with nutmeg and cracked black pepper.

Ladle the soup into bowls and pour some of the live yoghurt into each bowl to create a swirl pattern on the top. Sprinkle with nutmeg, serve with fresh rye bread and enjoy!

Green Veggie **Power Soup**

Serves 4

This is one amazing soup. The celery alone reduces acidity, which is beneficial in cases of arthritis, gout and stomach acidity. It's also a natural diuretic, helping to reduce fluid retention as well as balancing blood pH levels. Once you add the onion, broccoli, courgette, garlic, green beans, peas, asparagus and spinach, you have just about the ultimate power soup, which helps feed every cell in the body and flush out the waste.

60ml (2fl oz) olive oil
1 onion, finely chopped
2 garlic cloves, crushed
1 celery stick, chopped
1 courgette, chopped
1 head of broccoli, chopped
1.5 litres (2½ pints) vegetable stock
150g (5½oz) green beans, trimmed and chopped
150g (5½oz) green peas
150g (5½oz) asparagus, trimmed and cut into 1cm (½-inch) pieces
85g (3oz) baby spinach leaves, torn into pieces

Heat the olive oil in a large saucepan and cook the onion, garlic and celery until lightly browned. Add the courgette and broccoli and cook for 5 minutes.

Pour in the stock and bring to the boil. Simmer for 5 minutes then add the green beans, peas, asparagus and spinach. Continue to simmer for 5 minutes or until the vegetables are tender. Season well with cracked black pepper.

For extra taste, serve with a little dollop of home-made Pesto (page 249).

Carrot, Orange and Coriander
Soup

Serves 4

Coriander is packed with vitamins B, C and folic acid, plus potassium, sodium and magnesium. The essential oil in coriander stimulates the flow of bile and digestive juices as well as helping to relieve gas and stomach cramps. Add the carrot and orange and you have a wonderful-tasting, therapeutic and filling soup.

15g (½oz) organic butter
1 onion, peeled and finely chopped
455g (1lb) carrots, thinly sliced
700ml (1¼ pints) vegetable or chicken stock
1 tbsp (15ml) fresh coriander
Juice and pulp of 1 orange
Freshly ground black pepper
Chopped coriander to garnish

Melt the butter in a pan over a low heat. Stir in the onion and carrots and cook gently for 5 minutes. Add the remaining ingredients, cover the pan and cook gently for 30 minutes, until the carrots are soft. Allow the soup to cool slightly. Purée in a blender, return to the pan and reheat gently. Serve garnished with coriander.

Watercress and Baby Leek
Soup

Serves 4

As leeks are not for the juicer, using them in soup is a great way to obtain their goodness. This soup is rich, creamy, crammed with vitamins and minerals and, with the addition of 'live' yoghurt, also has some friendly bacteria to help keep the gut healthy.

55g (2oz) organic butter
2 sweet potatoes, peeled and roughly chopped
5 baby leeks, cleaned and chopped
115g (4oz) watercress, de-stalked and chopped
   (reserve a few leaves for garnish)
Freshly ground black pepper
850ml (1½ pints) vegetable stock
2 tbsp live yoghurt

Melt the butter in a heavy-based, lidded pan and add the sweet potatoes, leeks and watercress, making sure all the ingredients are covered with butter. Season with a little black pepper, put the lid on the pan and let the vegetables sweat over a very gentle heat for 20 minutes, giving it a little stir half-way through.

Add the stock, replace the lid and let everything simmer for a further 10–15 minutes or until the vegetables are quite soft. Let the mixture cool a little then transfer to a blender, give a good whiz and return to the saucepan. Stir in the live yoghurt, add a little more black pepper to taste if required and warm through gently.

Serve in soup bowls garnished with watercress leaves and a little more yoghurt swirled over the top. This soup can be served warm or cold depending on what you fancy!

Courgette and Dill **Soup**

Serves 4

If you have a cold, or you are just cold, then Nature's amazing antibiotics – in the form of garlic and onions – will soon lift you. It's also worth knowing that onions contain more calcium than any other food, so they are excellent for the teeth and bones. Once again, this super soup is packed with Nature's finest vitamins and minerals.

1–2 tbsp olive oil
1 small onion, chopped
1 garlic clove, crushed
455g (1lb) courgettes, roughly chopped
570–850ml (1–1½ pints) chicken or vegetable stock
1–3 tbsp finely chopped dill
Black pepper
Dill sprigs to garnish

Heat the oil in a saucepan and gently fry the onion and garlic until soft but not coloured. Add the courgettes and cook gently for 10–15 minutes until tender.

Add the stock, put the lid on the saucepan and simmer for a further 10–15 minutes.

Whiz the courgettes and a little stock in a blender until smooth. Bring to the boil with the remaining stock, dill and pepper.

Serve garnished with the dill sprigs.

Power
Lunches

During the programme I recommend having a Turbo Smoothie, a Turbo Salad or some Green Power Soup for lunch. However, not everyone will want a *pure* natural lunch every day after, or even during, the programme.

With that in mind I have put together some lunches you can get your teeth into, which will not compromise your health. The following recipes are loaded with many of the six dietary needs, and there's rarely a member of the seven deadly dietary sins to be found.

Although I have included these recipes in the lunch section, they all pretty much work for dinner too. Enjoy!

The Juice Master's
Turbo-power Sandwich

Serves 1

Not only delicious and incredibly filling, this also contains good-quality carbohydrates, fats and proteins, vitamins, minerals and the green plant food, chlorophyll. I often tuck into a version of this sandwich when I need something to get my teeth into at lunchtime rather than a smoothie or juice. Feel free to experiment and add your own ingredients, such as tomatoes, olives and different salad leaves.

2 slices German rye bread, toasted
Flesh of 1 ripe avocado
½ lemon
1 cup mixed baby leaf spinach and rocket leaves
¼ cup chopped spring onions
5 slices of organic cucumber
Organic mayonnaise
1 thin fillet cooked, lean, organic chicken breast or
   slice of cooked fish (any) or, if veggie, some tofu or Quorn
Freshly ground black pepper

Spread the freshly toasted rye bread with the avocado flesh. Add a dash of lemon juice on each side. Place the spinach and rocket on one slice of bread and add the spring onion and cucumber. Spread some mayonnaise over the chicken/fish/Quorn and place on top of the vegetables. Add black pepper and the remaining lemon juice and top with the other slice of bread. Cut in half before serving. If you can serve your choice of protein hot, then so much the better.

Chicken and Vegetable **Wraps**

Serves 2

A wonderful combination of healthy fats, natural water-rich carbohydrates and good-quality man-made carbohydrates. These wraps also contain friendly bacteria and lean protein, and are packed with vitamins and minerals. If you don't like an ingredient, simply leave it out! You may replace the chicken with fish, Quorn or tofu.

2 tbsp light soy sauce

¼ tsp Tabasco

2 boneless chicken breasts, skinned

1 small ripe avocado

1 tsp lemon/lime juice

1 tbsp chopped fresh chives

75ml (2½fl oz) live yoghurt

1 red pepper, seeds removed and cut into strips

8 button mushrooms

1 small red onion, quartered

4 wholemeal tortillas

Finely shredded lettuce, to serve

Put the soy and Tabasco sauces into a bowl and stir in the chicken. Cover and leave to stand for about 30 minutes, stirring occasionally.

Halve the avocado, remove the stone and scoop the flesh into a bowl. Squeeze the lemon/lime juice over the avocado and mash until smooth.

In another bowl, stir the chives into the yoghurt and mix well.

Arrange the chicken in the bottom tier of a steamer, and put the pepper, mushrooms and onion in the top tier. Next wrap the tortillas in foil, sealing well, and lay on top of the vegetables. Steam for 15 minutes until the chicken is cooked through, the vegetables are soft and the tortillas are warm. Cut the chicken into slices. Serve in separate dishes and tuck into whichever filling you fancy, topped with a little dollop of yoghurt and chive mix. You'll love it!

Jasey's
Veggie Sushi Rolls

Serves 2 as a snack or 1 as a meal

Don't let the word 'sushi' put you off – you won't find any raw fish around here!

These little rolls of veggie delight are packed with essential fats, protein, carbo-hydrates and antioxidants. They are much healthier than veggie sushi with white refined rice. That doesn't mean a trip to Yo Sushi is out of the question, but if you're going to make them yourself, make them as healthy as you can. The nori sheets, in case you were wondering, are seaweed – but don't let that put you off. They taste wonderful, contain vitamins A and C and have 0 per cent fat!

¼ cucumber
1 carrot
Flesh of 2 avocados
Raw nori sheets
1 onion, finely chopped
Few sprigs fresh dill

Prepare the cucumber and carrot by chopping into small, thin strips. Mash the avocado flesh and spread over the nori sheets, leaving a little space at one end to help seal the roll. Place a row of the cucumber, carrot, onion and dill down the centre of the nori sheets. Finally, roll the sheets from the bottom, ensuring you squeeze them tightly.

These are easy and great fun, and the filling can be changed to what-ever takes your fancy.

Great as a **snack** or a **meal** – best served **with soy sauce** and **chopsticks.**

Hemp/Spelt Pasta with Basil and
Tangy Lemon and Lime Sauce

Serves 2

Quick, easy, simple and flipping beautiful! Unlike wheat-based pasta, this lunchtime beauty won't make you feel bloated or fall asleep at your desk! Hemp and spelt pasta is now widely available.

Once again, feel free to adjust this power lunch to suit your tastes. A great alternative is simply to add some green pesto (page 249) to the pasta and serve with a small bowl of salad.

Packed with good-quality man-made carbohydrates, essential fatty acids, vitamins and minerals – and bursting with taste.

200g (7oz) hemp/spelt pasta
Juice of ½ lemon
Juice of ½ lime
1½ tbsp cold-pressed olive oil
¼ cup finely grated Parmesan cheese
½ cup small fresh basil leaves
¼ cup small olives, chopped
Cracked black pepper

Cook the pasta as per packet instructions until *al dente*. Place the lemon and lime juice and olive oil in a bowl and whisk together. Stir in the Parmesan, basil, olives and black pepper.

Drain the pasta and return to the warm saucepan, then toss with the sauce. Serve immediately.

The Juice Master's
Power Pittas

Serves 1

This is so tasty, simple and filling – and amazingly good for you.

Yes, it contains wheat and no, I'm not the biggest fan of the stuff. However, not everyone has a problem with wheat and, as I will emphasize until I'm blue in the face, the body can easily deal with small amounts of anything – including wheat. Wholemeal pittas are a great way of getting plenty of good stuff inside you as it's easy to pack them full of salad and other life-giving foods.

2 wholemeal pittas
1 ripe avocado
½ lemon/lime
1 tin of sardines
Handful of rocket, watercress and spinach leaves
Handful of alfalfa sprouts

Put the pittas under a grill and toast lightly. While they are toasting, stone the avocado and scoop out the flesh, mixing with a squeeze of lemon or lime juice.

Open the pittas and pack them with the avocado mix, sardines, rocket/watercress/spinach and alfalfa sprouts. Squeeze a little more lemon/lime juice over each and tuck in.

Hot Tip!
Wholemeal pittas can be stuffed with just about anything. All you need is a little imagination. You can have some hot fish, chicken, or whatever, stuffed with a load of freshly prepared salad, or some stir-fried veggies packed in with some green pesto. The options are almost limitless.

The Juice Master's
Protein Snack Attack

Serves 1

Other than a piece of fruit, this is probably the quickest and easiest lunch you can get. It is also packed with good fats and proteins, which will take the edge off any hunger. This recipe makes one portion, but provided you don't eat it with anything else except salad or veggies, you can have as much as you like!

2 (95g) tins boneless sardines in sunflower oil
Flesh of 1 large avocado
½ lemon

Simple – place the sardines and avocado flesh in a small bowl. Squeeze on the lemon juice, mix together and eat!

Hot Tip!
You can replace the sardines with mackerel, tuna or whatever you like, and you can add lime juice instead of lemon.

Herby Stuffed Peppers

Serves 4

One of those recipes you shouldn't knock until you've tried. Peppers are packed with beta-carotene, folic acid, potassium, vitamin C and phyto-nutrients, which all help prevent cardiovascular disease.

170g (6oz) couscous
300ml (½ pint) hot vegetable stock
1 tsp ground mixed spice
2 tbsp extra virgin olive oil
1 tbsp lemon juice
4 spring onions, thinly sliced
3 tbsp fresh parsley, finely chopped
3 tbsp fresh mint, finely chopped
Freshly ground black pepper
4 medium red, yellow or orange peppers

Put the couscous into a large bowl, pour over the hot vegetable stock and stir in the mixed spice. Leave to stand for about 5 minutes or until the stock has been absorbed. Stir in the oil, lemon juice, onions, herbs and black pepper to taste.

Cut tops off the peppers and remove the seeds. Spoon the couscous mixture into the peppers, press it in lightly and stand them in a steamer. You may need to trim the bottoms off the peppers to flatten them so they stand upright.

Steam for about 20 minutes or until peppers are soft.

The Juice Master's
Homemade Houmous with Pitta

Serves 1–2

Houmous – it may look like wallpaper paste, but it's actually OK on the health front. It's a good source of protein, and the wholemeal pittas aren't a bad form of carbohydrate, provided you can eat wheat. Houmous and warm pittas taste blooming good!

If making your own houmous is just too much grief, feel free to get some ready-made and add the other ingredients.

1 (440g) can chickpeas
1 garlic clove, roughly chopped
2 tsp toasted sesame oil or olive oil
2 tbsp lemon juice
Freshly ground black pepper
Chopped fresh parsley or coriander to serve
2 wholemeal pittas

Drain the chickpeas, reserving 2 tbsp of the juice. Put into a blender with the liquid and whiz. Add the garlic, oil and lemon juice and whiz again for about 30 seconds. Transfer to a serving bowl and season with pepper. Sprinkle with either the parsley or coriander.

Warm the pitta breads under the grill or lightly toast in a toaster and serve either whole or sliced to dip into the houmous.

Let's Do
Dinner

One of my key tips for losing weight – and keeping it off – is to have an evening meal free of 'man-made' carbohydrates such as pasta, potatoes and bread. However, for those OK on the weight front, or who need a little more variety, I have devised some dishes which do include some good-quality carbohydrates. Once again, I have made sure they are brimming with vitamins, minerals, essential fats and good proteins, and that they are high in natural water content to aid the digestive process.

Cooking isn't really rocket science, and you are welcome to adjust any of the recipes. If I have used chicken, for example, the meal usually works just as well with fish or a veggie alternative. In a fish recipe, you can swap the type of fish used to one you prefer. The key is not to get all steamed up with this cooking lark – just do what works for you and your lifestyle.

These recipes also work well for lunch. Let's tuck in!

Thyme for Tuna

Serves 2

Fresh tuna is in a different world to the poor excuse you find in a tin. It is loaded with essential fatty acids and is an excellent source of protein. When you throw in the other ingredients, you have a meal packed with calcium, vitamins C and E, lycopene, potassium and beta-carotene.

1 tbsp olive oil
1 tbsp lemon juice
1 clove garlic, crushed
2 tbsp thyme leaves
Freshly ground black pepper
2 tuna steaks
1 small red onion, sliced into thin rings
10 cherry tomatoes
6 green olives, sliced into rings

Mix together the olive oil, lemon juice, crushed garlic, thyme and black pepper. Pour into a shallow dish large enough to accommodate the fish. Add the tuna steaks, ensuring they are covered in the oil mixture, cover and leave to stand for 30 minutes or so.

Lay each tuna steak on a piece of baking paper or tin foil large enough to enclose it completely. Drizzle any remaining juices from the dish over the fish. Divide up the onion rings and place over the tuna. Add the tomatoes and olives. Close the parcel, leaving plenty of space around the contents and sealing the edges well.

Put the two parcels in a steamer and steam for about 12 minutes until the tuna is just cooked.

Oven-steamed Chicken and Vegetables

Serves 1

Once again, this nutrient-packed meal can be easily adapted to a fish-only or vegetarian diet. It's packed with iron, folic acid, potassium, vitamins A and C as well as good proteins, fats and carbohydrates.

55g (2oz) organic butter
1 piece of lean, organic, boneless chicken breast
Freshly ground black pepper
1 lemon
1 clove garlic, crushed
100g (4oz) broccoli
55g (2oz) cauliflower
½ sweet potato, peeled
1 carrot, topped and tailed
1 courgette, topped and tailed
55g (2oz) flat-leaf parsley, chopped

Preheat the oven to 220°C/425°F/Gas Mark 7. Rub the butter over the chicken breast and season with black pepper. Squeeze over a little of the lemon and add the crushed garlic. Put the chicken in some tin foil and scrunch into a pocket, leaving a little 'air room' for steaming. Put in the oven for 15–20 minutes.

Steam all the vegetables for 10 minutes or so or until cooked to your preference. Remove the chicken from the oven, put on a serving plate and pour some of the remaining juice over it. Put the vegetables onto the plate as well, and pop the remaining butter over them. Add a little more black pepper, squeeze the remaining juice over everything and garnish with chopped parsley.

Honey-glazed Vegetables

Serves 2

This recipe is just great for a cold winter's night. This dish contains vitamins B, C and K, lycopene, which has anti-cancer properties, calcium, iron, silicon, potassium, phosphorous and iodine. The sweet potato provides beta-carotene and is excellent for building body strength.

1 red onion
2 sweet potatoes
3 carrots, topped and tailed
6 baby tomatoes
1 courgette, topped and tailed
2 parsnips, topped and tailed
2 garlic cloves, halved
3 tbsp organic Manuka honey
Lemon juice
Ground black pepper

Preheat the oven to a low setting (150°C/300°F/Gas Mark 2) so the vegetables don't burn on the outside and remain hard on the inside.

Prepare the vegetables by scrubbing where possible and peeling as necessary. Cut into hefty chunks and place in a big roasting tray. Dot the garlic cloves around the vegetables. Mix the honey with the lemon juice and drizzle over the vegetables, tossing them to ensure they are all covered, and season with black pepper. Cover the roasting tray with tin foil for the first hour of cooking and uncover for the last 15 minutes to crisp the vegetables up a little. Keep a close eye, though, to ensure the vegetables don't burn.

Cook for about 1¼ hours or until the vegetables are soft when you pierce with a sharp knife.

This is a meal in itself, but if you feel like something extra serve with some lovely rye bread spread with avocado and lemon juice, or some fish like mackerel or salmon.

Jasey's
Fish Kebabs with Pineapple and Steamed Veggies

Serves 1

This really is delicious and, again, extremely good for you. The pineapple contains an enzyme called bromelain, which helps to digest the proteins in the fish. The steamed veggies supply the finest vitamins, minerals and carbohydrates from Nature's pharmacy. If you are on the 14-day plan, I would highly recommend this for dinner on more than one occasion.

1 x 285g (10oz) swordfish steak
Cold-pressed olive oil
Balsamic vinegar
Juice of 1 lemon
2 cups broccoli
4 asparagus spears
⅓ small pineapple, peeled and cubed
Freshly ground black pepper

Preheat the grill to its highest setting. Brush the fish lightly with olive oil and balsamic vinegar and place on a tray in the middle of the grill. Cook for 3 minutes on each side then lower the heat to medium. Squeeze the lemon juice over the fish and cook for a further 3 minutes on each side. Remove and cut fish into cubes.

Steam the broccoli for 8–10 minutes and the asparagus for 2 minutes.

To make the kebabs, put the cubes of pineapple and fish alternately on to a skewer. You should end up with three skewers of kebabs. Place skewers under a hot grill for 2 minutes, turning them after a minute.

Place the broccoli and asparagus on the plate, spread with butter and sprinkle with pepper. Lay the skewers over the veggies and serve.

Rice with Red Lentils

Serves 4–6 (adjust amounts accordingly for fewer portions)

Umm ... rice and lentils – almost makes you want to get naked and climb a tree! Despite the 'hippy' image, lentils are even more efficient complete protein providers than meat, but without the fat! They also have B vitamins, calcium and iron. If lentils give you gas, please do yourself and your friends a favour – swap them for some fish, chicken or other veggie alternative that doesn't come from the bean family!

1 tbsp coriander seeds
1 tbsp cardamom pods
1 tbsp cumin seeds
1 tsp whole black peppercorns
1 tsp whole cloves
1 small cinnamon stick, crushed
60ml (2fl oz) olive oil
1 onion, chopped
3 garlic cloves, chopped
255g (9oz) red lentils
200g (7oz) basmati rice
750ml (3 cups) hot vegetable stock
Spring onion, sliced diagonally, to garnish

Place all the spices in a dry frying pan and shake over a medium heat for 1 minute, or until fragrant. Blend to a fine powder in a spice grinder or blender. Heat the olive oil in a thick-based saucepan. Add the onion, garlic and 3 tsp of the powdered spice mix. Cook over a medium heat for 3 minutes, or until the onion is browning and soft.

Stir in the lentils and rice and cook for 2 minutes. Add the stock and stir well. Slowly bring to the boil, then reduce the heat and simmer with the lid on for 15–20 minutes, or until the rice is cooked and all the stock has been absorbed. Gently fluff the rice with a fork and garnish with spring onion.

The Juice Master's
Fish 'n' Chips

Serves 1–2

This is a brilliant alternative to the usual version of this great British dish. The main reason for this is that it's actually good for you! Packed with vitamins, minerals, essential fatty acids, antioxidants and an abundance of beautiful flavours, it's not only wonderful on the health front, but tastes amazing.

2 medium sweet potatoes, sliced lengthways
Olive oil
1 small red onion, chopped
A handful of mixed herbs (e.g. parsley, thyme, basil), finely chopped
1 clove garlic, chopped
Freshly ground black pepper
1½ cups runner beans
10–14 oz cod steak
1 lemon
Organic butter
A handful of pine nuts

Preheat the oven to 220ºC/425ºF/Gas Mark 7. Place a piece of greaseproof paper in a baking tray and rub it with olive oil. Brush the sweet potatoes with some olive oil and place in the baking tray along with the garlic, onion, pine nuts and half the herbs. Season well with black pepper. Bake in the middle of the oven for 15 minutes.

Turn over the sliced potatoes, add the runner beans and pour over some more olive oil. Place the fish in with the beans and potatoes and add the rest of the herbs and a squeeze of lemon juice. Lightly cover the baking tray with tin foil and cook for another 15 minutes.

To serve, arrange the cod and potato herb mixture on a plate and add more lemon juice and a knob of butter. Enjoy!

Juicy Stir-fried
Monkfish 'n' Veggie Special

Serves 1–2

This is extremely quick and easy to make and, considering it's super-fast food, it's packed with goodness. In this juicy stir-fry you'll find vitamins B and C, folic acid and beta-carotene and the minerals calcium, iron, zinc, sodium, manganese, phosphorous, silicon and selenium. The fennel has a calming effect on digestion, reducing intestinal gas, flatulence and bloating. Red onions are the richest dietary source of quercetin, a potent antioxidant and cancer-inhibiting phytochemical. Once you take into account the amino acids, the natural carbohydrates, the high water content and the fish which is a good source of protein, you have one of the finest nutritional meals on the planet – enjoy and always be grateful for the food choices you have on a daily basis.

If you are doing the Turbo-charge programme this meal fits perfectly into your evening meal choices.

Juicy 10 oz piece of monkfish, diced into cubes
   or strips (your choice)
½ cup diced organic carrot
½ orange bell pepper, diced
½ yellow bell pepper, diced
A small handful of mangetout
½ cup diced red onion
½ cup broccoli florets
½ cup diced courgette
¼ cup diced fennel
½ lemon
½ lime
Dash of cold pressed virgin olive oil
Dash of freshly ground black pepper

Use a wok for this recipe if you have one – if not, a normal frying pan will do.

Put a dash of olive oil into the wok and blast up the heat. Once the oil is hot, throw in the monkfish and toss for 3–4 minutes. Chuck in the diced courgette, fennel, carrot and peppers along with the broccoli and mangetout. Toss all these ingredients together and cook for a further 6–8 minutes, or until the fish is properly cooked through.

Place in a bowl and drizzle a little olive oil over the lot. Squeeze the lemon and lime juice over everything and add a pinch of freshly ground pepper – beautiful!

Steam
Cuisine

Salmon with Vegetable Courgette

Serves 2

This is a great way to liven up some vegetables and present them in an enticing way for all the family to enjoy. It's loaded with calcium, essential fatty acids, beta-carotene, folic acid, potassium and wonderful phyto-chemicals that help prevent blood clots, strokes and heart disease.

1 medium courgette
1 small red or orange pepper, halved and deseeded
1 spring onion
2 skinless salmon fillets
Freshly ground black pepper
½ lemon
2 knobs organic butter
2 dill sprigs

Using a vegetable peeler, cut the courgette lengthways into long, thin strands, and cut the pepper into long, thin strips.

Half the onion crossways then cut each piece lengthways into quarters to make thin strips.

Put the salmon fillets on separate pieces of baking paper or foil, large enough to enclose them completely with a little room left. Scatter the vegetables over the salmon and season with black pepper. Sprinkle with lemon juice, then put a knob of butter and a sprig of dill on each fillet. Close the parcels, leaving plenty of space around the contents.

Arrange the two parcels in a steamer and steam for 6–8 minutes or until the fish is cooked.

Foiled Fish

Serves 2

The idea with this one is to chuck everything in some tin foil and let it do the work for you! It's quick, easy and very tasty. It's also stupidly good for you and perfect as a dinner on the 14-day plan and beyond. The asparagus alone contains vitamins B and C, folic acid and the anti-cancer king, beta-carotene. It's loaded with the minerals calcium, iron, phosphorous, magnesium and potassium – and that's before you get to the other ingredients.

2 undyed cod/haddock loin steaks
1 red pepper
1 yellow pepper
½ red onion
Handful of mangetout
5 baby corn
5 baby tomatoes
5 asparagus spears
½ lemon, ½ lime

Preheat the oven to 180°C/350°F/Gas Mark 4. Place the fish on a piece of tin foil large enough to make an envelope for the fish with room to spare. Prepare the vegetables by deseeding and slicing the peppers and slicing the onion to your preferred size. Then, basically, throw everything in with the fish. Squeeze lemon and lime juice over the fish and vegetables, and put a couple of wedges of each in the envelope as well. Season with black pepper.

Fold the tin foil over the fish and vegetables, making sure it is sealed. Place in a baking tin and cook for 20–25 minutes. The fish is ready when it flakes away nicely when tested with a fork. Transfer to a serving plate and pour over the juice in the tin foil pocket – this is absolutely delicious and tastes almost like a clear soup. If you need a little something else, avocado is a lovely addition with some lemon juice squeezed over.

Salsa **Salmon**

Serves 2

Packed with beta-carotene, lycopene, potassium, vitamins C and E, calcium, good fats and excellent proteins, it tastes flipping good too!

Freshly ground black pepper
2 salmon steaks
10 cherry tomatoes
2 sun-blushed or sun-dried tomatoes in oil,
  drained and finely chopped
2 spring onions, thinly sliced
2 tsp olive oil
2 tsp balsamic vinegar
½ tsp organic Manuka honey
8–10 fresh basil leaves

Sprinkle black pepper over both sides of the salmon and press it in well. Arrange the fish on a sheet of baking paper in a steamer.

Mix all the ingredients together, apart from the basil leaves, in a bowl that will fit in the steamer. Cover the bowl with foil, sealing around the edges, and place in the steamer as well.

Steam everything for about 8 minutes or until the fish is cooked.

Tear up the basil leaves and stir them into the tomato mixture. Place the salmon on a serving plate and top with the lovely tomato salsa. Season if you wish with more freshly ground black pepper. Enjoy.

Citrus **Snapper**

Serves 2

Not only does it taste incredible, but once again nutrition is high on the list. This 'snappy' dish is packed with anti-cancer carotenoids as well as good fats, and an array of vitamins and minerals including folic acid, magnesium, potassium and vitamin A.

125g (4½oz) organic carrots
125g (4½oz) organic courgettes
1 tsp caraway seeds
2 x 170g (6oz) snapper fillets
1 orange, unpeeled
2 tbsp cold-pressed olive oil
½ bunch coriander, roughly chopped

Cut the carrots and courgettes into long, diagonal slices and place into a hot, lightly oiled grill pan. Cook for 3 minutes on each side, sprinkling the caraway seeds over the vegetables for the last 2 minutes. Remove from the pan and keep warm.

Cook the snapper in the same lightly oiled pan for 3 minutes on each side.

While the fish is cooking, cut the orange into quarters and cook 2 of the quarters in a pan until the flesh sides are charred.

Squeeze the juice from the remaining orange quarters and mix well with the olive oil.

Reserve some of the chopped coriander for decoration and add the rest to the carrots and courgettes, mixing together.

Place the carrots and courgettes on a serving plate and put the snapper on top. Pour over the orange and oil dressing and sprinkle with the remaining chopped coriander.

Dips

The following are great additions to meals or are superb on their own as 'dips'.

Cut vegetables into strips or warm some wholemeal pittas or strips of rye bread and simply dip and eat.

Roasted Aubergine **Dip**

Serves 1–2

Great served with freshly cut veggies or some warm strips of German rye bread. The fresh coriander, lemon, chilli and spring onion really add some zing to what can be the rather dull taste of aubergine.

Aubergines contain anthocyanins, particularly nasuin, which are powerful antioxidants. They also contain folate, potassium and fibre.

1 large aubergine
1 tsp soy sauce
1 tsp sweet chilli sauce
½ tsp lemon juice
1 tbsp fresh coriander, chopped
2 spring onions, finely sliced

Preheat the oven to 200°/400°F/Gas Mark 6. Cut the aubergine in half lengthways and score the flesh with a sharp knife. Place in the oven on a baking sheet and cook for 30 minutes.

Leave to cool then scrape away the flesh from the skin – the skin can then be discarded.

Place the flesh in a food processor or blender with the soy sauce, chilli sauce and lemon juice. Blitz until smooth.

Mix in the coriander and sliced spring onion and serve with crudités of carrot and celery. Again, lightly toasted wholemeal pitta breads are great dipped into this.

Great **Guacamole**

This recipe is one of my favourites. Guacamole is incredibly versatile and a great source of essential fat. It makes a great dip with raw vegetables or as a spread on sandwiches.

Flesh of 1 large avocado
1 large plum tomato
1 tbsp fresh coriander
1 tbsp fresh parsley
1 garlic clove
½ red chilli
Juice of 1 lemon

Roughly chop the avocado and tomato. Blend everything together, except the lemon juice, in a blender. When smooth, add the lemon juice and blend for a further minute or so or until the mixture starts to thicken. Serve with whichever accompaniment you wish and enjoy.

Butter Dip

Serves 2–4

½ cup plain live yoghurt
⅓ cup nut butter
3 tbsp lemon juice
1½ tbsp chopped fresh parsley
1 small garlic clove
¼ tsp ground cumin
Several dashes of cayenne pepper

Mix all the ingredients together thoroughly with a fork or whisk, or whiz in a blender. This dip is great served with raw or steamed vegetables.

Jasey's **Sassy Salsa**

Serves 1–2

This salsa works really well if all the ingredients are cut into fairly beefy chunks. It gives it a great texture to go with its lovely vibrant colour. Great with warm pittas, or if you are having a 'keeping it real' moment, with tortilla chips!

1 red pepper, deseeded and chopped
1 chilli, deseeded and chopped
3 plum tomatoes, chopped
½ red onion, chopped
Squeeze of lime juice
Black pepper
Coriander leaves, chopped

Throw everything together in a bowl, mix thoroughly, season and enjoy!

Pesto

Pesto is an extremely versatile dip. It's great on its own with pasta or as an amazing sauce on fish, chicken or freshly prepared salad. Also wonderful mixed in with The Juice Master's Turbo-power Sandwich (page 224).

½ cup pine nuts
1 cup fresh basil leaves or herb/leaves of your choice
1 clove of garlic, diced
2 tbsp olive oil
Pinch of sea salt

Simple – just pound all the ingredients together using a pestle and mortar. If you don't have a pestle and mortar, simply put all the ingredients into a cup and mix, remembering to dice the basil leaves.

How to Make a Juice – Fast

1. Get all the ingredients you need on your chopping board.
2. Prepare, wash and cut to size the produce you need for your juice and put back the rest.
3. Half-fill the sink with warm water and washing-up liquid.
4. Turn on the machine and juice everything in one go.
5. Put the jug of juice to one side and begin cleaning.
6. Scrape bits off the chopping board onto newspaper and wash the board immediately.
7. Undo the machine and lift out any pulp in nooks and crannies and place on newspaper.
8. Put all parts of machine (except electric base) into the sink of warm water.
9. Fold the newspaper and throw in bin or empty contents in garden and paper in bin.
10. Run tap with warm water and keep it running.
11. Most pieces of the machine can be cleaned simply by rinsing them under the tap. The mesh part will need the nail brush and tap treatment.
12. Quickly run a tea towel over the machine, put it back together and leave everything in a position where it's once again inviting and easy to juice.

Appendix

VITAMINS	BENEFITS	SOURCE
Vitamin A	Helps maintain healthy skin, eyes and bones Boosts healthy immune system Essential for development and growth of cells	Dark green leafy vegetables like broccoli, watercress, spinach, kale, beet greens and deep orange fruits and vegetables like carrots, oranges, apricots, papayas and mangoes
Beta-carotene	Converted by body into Vitamin A as needed Powerful antioxidant Helps promote faster healing of mucous membranes Good for cardiovascular health Stimulates immune system Healthy skin	Carrots, kale, spinach, parsley, chard, beet greens, watercress, mangoes, cantaloupes, apricots, broccoli, pumpkin, watermelon, asparagus
Thiamin (Vitamin B1)	Involved in release of energy from carbohydrates Important for brain and nerves which use glucose for their energy needs	Yeast, yeast extracts, pork, wholegrain cereals (brown rice, wholemeal bread), nuts and pulses, green vegetables
Vitamin B2 (Riboflavin)	Needed for production of energy from food Aids normal growth of body tissues Healthy skin and vision Needed for healthy nerve function	Kale, parsley, broccoli, beet greens, prunes, asparagus, avocados, almonds
Vitamin B3 (Niacin)	Releases energy from food Aids in maintenance of skin Brain and nerve function Proper mental functioning	Brewer's yeast (dried), tempeh, broad beans, peas, peanuts, brown rice, soya beans, wheat bran, red pepper, spring greens, dried peaches, wholemeal bread, oily fish

VITAMINS	BENEFITS	SOURCE
Vitamin B6 (Pyridoxine)	Helps form red blood cells Important in maintaining healthy nervous system Important in healthy brain functioning Helps body build all types of cells, hormones and anti-bodies Anti-anxiety vitamin – especially for women	Kale, spinach, turnip greens, peppers, cauliflowers, prunes, avocados, bananas, carrots, hazelnuts, salmon, soybeans, sunflower seeds, tuna, wheatgerm
Vitamin B12 (Cobalamin)	Normal cell growth and development Prevents pernicious anaemia Healthy nervous system	Eggs, oily fish, seaweed, cheese, soya milks
Vitamin C	Helps increase activity of white blood cells which are foremost cells in immune system helping resistance against infections Keeps tissues strong and healthy Helps sweep up damaging free radicals Helps with wound healing Aids body's absorption of iron and calcium	Blackcurrants, strawberries, kiwi, broccoli, Brussels sprouts, grapefruit, peppers, kale, lemons, oranges, papayas, spinach, tomatoes, watercress and guavas
Vitamin D	Helps control use of calcium, needed for strong bones and teeth Healthy joints	Cold-water fish such as herring, mackerel, salmon and sardines, sunflower seeds
Vitamin E	Helps protect skin Can relax smooth muscles of airways Helps brain from free radical attack Repairs tissues Antioxidant that helps immune system Helps growth and repair of inner lining of arterial walls Normalizes abnormal hormone levels Anti-inflammatory Promotes healing and aids in reducing levels of stomach acid Improves circulation	Spinach, watercress, asparagus, carrots, tomatoes, almonds, hazelnuts, sunflower seeds, wheatgerm
Vitamin K	Blood clotting	Spinach, broccoli, kale, cabbage, Brussels sprouts, dried seaweed
Folic Acid	Great for blood cells Prevention of birth defects Protects against anaemia	Brewer's yeast (dried), green leafy vegetables, citrus fruits, eggs, dried fruits, nuts, oats, pulses, wheat germ

MINERALS	BENEFITS	SOURCE
Calcium	Vital for strong bones and teeth Needed for muscles to contract and relax properly Healthy nerve function	Brazil nuts, cheese, greens, yoghurt, chickpeas, tinned sardines, milk
Chromium	Key component of glucose tolerance factor (GTF) which works with insulin to regulate blood-sugar levels	Potato, green pepper, apple, parsnip, banana, spinach, carrot, wholemeal bread, wheatgerm
Copper	Involved in the making of red blood cells Production of bone and general body tissue maintenance Also important for various chemicals in nervous system	Nuts, peas, beans, cereals, brown rice, sunflower seeds, chickpeas, dried pineapple, sesame seeds
Iodine	Needed for proper function of thyroid gland and production of thyroid hormones	Fish, seaweeds
Iron	Prevents anaemia Helps produce haemoglobin which carries oxygen around the body	Green leafy vegetables, dried fruits, wholemeal bread, lentils, legumes, nuts, sesame and pumpkin seeds, chickpeas
Magnesium	Essential for healthy bones and teeth Plays an important part in our enzyme systems that help us make use of energy in our tissues Needed to help Vitamins B1 and B6 work efficiently Transmits nerve impulses Important in muscle contraction	Brazil nuts, almonds, cashews, sunflower seeds, sesame seeds, butternut squash, soya-based protein, soya beans, spinach, bananas, brown rice, wheat bran
Manganese	Important for healthy cell function Proper bone development Efficient protein and fat metabolism	Most fruits and vegetables, whole grains, nuts, brown rice, wholemeal spaghetti, pine nuts, blackberries, bananas, curly kale, sweet potatoes, wheat-bran
Phosphorous	Plays vital role in the release and use of energy from food Also important building block for various proteins, carbohydrates and fats	Brown rice, tempeh, tahini paste, peas, beans, lentils, nuts, seeds, tofu, sweet potato, Brussels sprouts, rye flour, spring greens

MINERALS	BENEFITS	SOURCE
Potassium	Important for maintaining fluid balance Proper muscle and nerve function Involved in maintaining normal blood-sugar levels Helps control blood pressure	Bananas, avocado, potatoes, sweet potatoes, fresh fruit, dried fruits, nuts, spinach, courgette, Brussels sprouts, spring greens, Swiss chard, butter beans, soya beans, wholemeal bread
Selenium	Proper function of red blood cells Powerful antioxidant Protects against heart disease	Brazil nuts, lentils, wholemeal flour, sunflower seeds, red kidney beans, soya beans, walnuts, dried apricots and peaches, celery, tuna, white fish, sardines
Sodium	Important for maintaining correct amount of fluid in body Plays a vital role in both nerve and muscle function	Olives, vine leaves, rye bread, Swiss chard, spinach, pistachio nuts, celeriac
Zinc	Component of insulin; required for blood-sugar control Needed for proper taste and hearing Important in wound healing and enzyme activation Male fertility Growth Hormone function Liver function Immunity	Lentils, peas, dried seaweed, seeds, pine nuts, wholemeal bread, wheat germ, pecan nuts, cashew nuts, chickpeas

HERBivores

Herbs are a very natural and logical ingredient in some of the recipes in this book. They are not only incredibly easy to take, but they have amazing healing properties that will benefit many an ailment and also generally boost your overall well-being.

The great news is that all of these herbs, whether you have heard of them or not, are readily available in most good health shops in an easy-to-use form. The following very-quick-at-a-glance table outlines the uses of herbs and the forms in which they can be obtained.

HERB	USE	AVAILABLE FORMS
Basil	Memory and stimulates nerve and brain cells	Leaves
Echinacea	Great for boosting immune system and warding off colds and germs	Tincture, tablets
Garlic	Member of the lily family Strengthens immune system Antibacterial and antibiotic Lowers blood pressure Blood cholesterol Cancer-preventing Raw garlic more powerful than cooked	Fresh bulb, dried
Ginger	Stimulant that encourages sweating to eliminate toxins and dispels catarrh, hence great for colds Aids digestion Reduces nausea and motion sickness	Root, dried extract
Gingko biloba	Great for maintaining brain function Oxygenates blood Helps to increase mental alertness, memory and concentration Helps blood flow AVOID IF PREGNANT	Extract, dried leaf or tablet
Ginseng	This herb helps to detoxify the body. It is anti-fatigue and anti-stress Tonic and mental stimulant	Root, extract, capsule, tea

HERB	USE	AVAILABLE FORMS
Lavender	Relaxing Comfort to the stomach	Oil, dried, tablet
Milk thistle	A potent antioxidant and liver detoxifier	Extract, powder
Nutmeg	Anti-inflammatory Relieves muscle spasms Relaxes stomach muscles, good for wind and cramps Sedative DO NOT USE WHEN PREGNANT	Dried kernel
Parsley	Historically used for a diuretic, tonic and a help to digestion problems It can help to encourage menstruation and stimulate milk flow Rich in Vitamins A and C, iron, calcium, magnesium and manganese AVOID OR HAVE SMALL AMOUNTS IF PREGNANT	Fresh leaves, dried
Peppermint	Aids digestion Very uplifting Powerful antiseptic in its oil form Peppermint tea great for relief of colds and flu	Fresh leaves, oil, tea
Thyme	Antiseptic Antibiotic Great for colds, flu and all respiratory infections Useful for cystitis Good mouthwash for gum problems	Fresh leaves, dried

INGREDIENT BENEFITS

Alfalfa sprouts Contains folic acid, zinc, calcium, silicon, Vitamins A, B complex, C, E and K. A diuretic and a stimulant

Apple Vitamins A, B and C, potassium, pectin, boron, ellagic acid, carotenes. A great system cleanser, full of dietary fibre, laxative, lowers cholesterol

Apricots Beta-carotene, potassium, boron, iron, magnesium, fibre, Vitamins A and C. May help with heart disease, normalize blood pressure and heart function

Artichoke Insulin, phosphorous, iron. A great stimulant for the immune system, great for detoxifying, may help lower blood pressure

Asparagus Vitamins A, C and E, potassium, niacin, iron, phosphorous, riboflavin, folic acid. A great antioxidant, diuretic and promotes healing

Avocado Potassium, essential fatty acids, Vitamins A, B, C and E, riboflavin, iron, calcium, copper, phosphorous, zinc, niacin, magnesium, folic acid. A great antioxidant and one of the most energy-dense fruits

Banana Potassium, fibre, Vitamins A, C and B6, folic acid, magnesium. A great immune booster, helps lower cholesterol and anti-bacterial

Beetroot Vitamins A, B and C folate, potassium, manganese. Leafy tops contain calcium, beta-carotene and iron. Thought to be anti-bacterial, antioxidant, tonic, cleansing and a laxative

Blackberries Vitamins C and E, fibre, potassium, iron, calcium, manganese, beta-carotene, phosphorous. Beneficial for heart and circulatory problems

Blackcurrants Vitamin C, potassium, calcium, magnesium, phosphorous. Anti-inflammatory and cancer-fighting phytochemicals. Anti-bacterial, immune enhancer, promotes healing, anti-diarrhoea

Blueberries Beta-carotene, Vitamin C, calcium, magnesium, phosphorous, tannins (help kill viruses and bacteria), antioxidants. Great anti-bacterial fruit, antiviral, disease-fighting, anti-ageing

Broccoli Vitamins A, B, C and E, cancer-fighting phytochemicals, folic acid, iron, potassium, riboflavin. Good antioxidant and promotes healing

Cabbage Vitamins C and E, cancer-fighting phytochemicals, beta-carotene, folic acid, iron, potassium. Powerful antioxidant, cleanser, immune builder, anti-bacterial, helps memory, diuretic, anti-inflammatory and antiseptic

Carrots Beta-carotene, Vitamins A, B and C, folic acid, magnesium, potassium, iron, calcium. They have a cleansing effect on the liver and digestive system. Great antioxidant, anti-cancer, antiseptic, diuretic, immune booster, anti-bacterial, helps lower blood cholesterol, aids eye and skin problems

Cauliflower Vitamin C, potassium, protein, iron, anti-cancer, antioxidant

Celery Potassium, calcium, Vitamin C. Anti-bacterial, great cleanser, calms and rebuilds red blood cells

Chard Calcium, cancer-fighting phytochemicals, carotenes, iron, phosphorous, Vitamins A and C. A great antioxidant

Cherries Ellagic Acid (anti-cancer agent), Vitamins A and C, biotin, potassium, folic acid, beta-carotene, calcium, flavonoids, magnesium. Packed with pectin – soluble fibre that helps control blood cholesterol levels and a great anti-bacterial

INGREDIENT BENEFITS

Chicory	Folic acid, potassium, iron, potassium, Vitamin A. It stimulates appetite and cleanses the digestive system
Chilli pepper	Vitamins A and C, calcium, iron, magnesium, phosphorous, potassium. Positive effect on blood cholesterol, stimulant, tonic, antiseptic, anti-bacterial, relieves mucous, decongestant, stomach muscle relaxer
Cranberries	Vitamins A and C, iodine, calcium, beta-carotene, folic acid, chlorine, magnesium, phosphorous, potassium. Great for soothing the digestive and urinary tracts
Cucumber	Folic acid, calcium, chlorine, Vitamins B1, 2, 3 5 and 6, iron, potassium, beta-carotene. Highly diuretic, cleansing and great for hair, skin and nails. Also may help to reduce cholesterol
Fennel	Vitamins A, B6 and C, potassium, calcium. Cleanses digestive tract, great antioxidant, diuretic and a stimulant
Figs	Folic acid, beta-carotene, calcium, iron, potassium. Cleanses digestive tract, anti-bacterial, anti-cancer, laxative
Grapefruit	Beta-carotene, calcium, potassium, Vitamin C. Great cleansing juice, blood thinner and lowers cholesterol
Grapes	Vitamins C and E, calcium, antioxidants, phosphorous, flavonoids, potassium. Anti-cancer, good for clearing skin and digestive system
Horseradish	Vitamin C, phtyochemicals. Good antiobiotic
Kale	Beta-carotene, calcium, Vitamins A and C, chlorophyll, folic acid, iron, phosphorous. Anti-cancer and good antioxidants
Kiwi	Beta-carotene, Vitamins C and E, fibre, potassium. Antioxidant, anti-cancer, aids digestion, excellent cleanser and energizer
Leek	Beta-carotene, Vitamins A and C, folic acid, calcium. Diuretic, laxative, antiseptic, digestive, anti-arthritic, anti-inflammatory
Lemon	Vitamin C, beta-carotene, calcium, magnesium, bioflavonoids, potassium. Antioxidant, cleansing for liver and kidneys
Lettuce	Folic acid, potassium, Vitamins A, B6 and C. Juice is detoxifying and calming
Lime	Beta-carotene, folic acid, Vitamin C, calcium, potassium, bioflavonoids
Mango	Vitamins B and C, beta-carotene, flavonoids, potassium, antioxidants, magnesium. Anti-cancer
Melon	Vitamins A and C, calcium, folic acid, potassium, magnesium, phosphorous. Juice is cleansing and diuretic
Nectarine	Vitamin C, folic acid, calcium, magnesium, beta-carotene, potassium. Antioxidant, anti-cancer and energizing
Onion	Quercetin – a potent antioxidant. Anti-bacterial, anti-cancer, antioxidant, circulatory, digestive stimulant, lowers cholesterol
Orange	Calcium, folic acid, iron, potassium, thiamine, Vitamins B6 and C. Antioxidant, lowers blood cholesterol
Papaya	Beta-carotene, Vitamin C, calcium, magnesium. Antioxidant, energizes and cleanses the digestive tract

INGREDIENT BENEFITS

Parsnip Vitamins C and E, potassium, iron, calcium, folic acid. Anti-inflammatory, anti-cancer

Passionfruit Beta-carotene, phytochemicals, Vitamin C, magnesium. Antiseptic, sedative and slightly laxative

Peach Vitamins A, B3 and C, beta-carotene, flavonoids, potassium, niacin, iron. Antioxidant, anti-cancer

Pear Vitamin C, potassium, fibre. Juice helps protect the colon

Peppers Beta-carotene, folic acid, Vitamin C, calcium. Antioxidant, anti-cancer, heart protective, cleanses system and great for hair, nails and skin

Pineapple Potassium, Vitamin C, iron, folic acid. Juice cleanses intestines, helpful and helps boost the immune system

Plum Vitamins A, C and E, calcium, folic acid. Anti-bacterial, antioxidant, aids digestion, boosts immune system and stimulates appetite

Pomegranate Beta-carotene, Vitamin E, potassium. Anti-diarrhoea and heart protective

Prunes Beta-carotene, fibre, iron, niacin, potassium, Vitamin B6. Laxative

Pumpkin Folic acid, potassium, Vitamins A and C

Radish Iron, magnesium, potassium, iron. Stimulates gall bladder, heals mucous membranes

Raspberry Potassium, niacin, iron, Vitamin C, fibre. Great immunity enhancer

Rocket Folate, calcium, beta-carotene, Vitamin C

Spinach Beta-carotene, chlorophyll, folic acid, iron, choline, Vitamins A, C and E. Anti-cancer, helps memory, antioxidant, anti-anaemia

Spring onion Vitamins A and C, folic acid, potassium. Diuretic, anti-arthritic and anti-inflammatory

Squash Potassium, Vitamins A and C, folic acid. Anti-oxidant and anti-cancer

Strawberries Vitamins C and E, ellagic acid, folic acid, beta-carotene, potassium, iron. Antioxidant, anti-viral, anti-cancer, effective against gout, rheumatism and arthritis. Great cleansing juice and good liver tonic

Sweet potato Beta-carotene, Vitamins C, B6 and E, manganese, potassium. Excellent source of fibre with skin left on

Tomato Beta-carotene, lycopene, potassium, Vitamins C and E. Anti-cancer, antioxidant, helps maintain mental and physical functioning, relaxant

Turnip Calcium, iron, protein. Great tonic, decongestant, anti-bacterial, anti-cancer, diuretic, helps purify blood

Watercress Beta-carotene, iron, Vitamins A, C and E, potassium. Diuretic, cleanses intestines, stimulates appetite, antibiotic

Watermelon Folic acid, potassium, Vitamins A and C, iron, beta-carotene, calcium, magnesium, phosphorous. Cleansing diuretic, anti-bacterial, anti-cancer

For information on the Juice Master's DVDs, other books, health retreats, stop smoking programme, quit alcohol programme, the best juice extractors – plus anything else you need to know:

Call the Juice Master Hotline on 0044 845 130 28 29
(This is a UK number)
Websites: www.juicemaster.com   www.thejuicemaster.com
Email: info@thejuicemaster.com

Turbo-charge Your Life in 14 Days CD and DVD box set – a unique opportunity to have Jason Vale coach you through the entire 14 days using 14 individual CDs. This programme looks at every aspect of your health and life. If you want to lose weight, gain weight, reshape your body, increase your energy, change your eating and drinking patterns, stop smoking, cut down on or quit alcohol, or you simply need the ultimate, no-nonsense kick up the arse, then this programme is for you. The CDs go into much more detail than this book; they also contain Jason's other books and his Stop Smoking in 2 Hours CD programme. Available 2006 – to be put on the waiting list please send an email to boxset@thejuicemaster.com

The Juice Master's Mind and Body Detox Retreats – a truly amazing experience. You spend a week in a beautiful European or US coastal destination, drinking the finest-quality freshly extracted juices, eating beautiful natural foods, doing yoga, playing games, having wonderful walks and runs, meeting new people and attending seminars designed to change the way you think about feeding yourself. There isn't enough time here to get a full picture of this amazing week, so please get on the website, see for yourself and read the following comments to get a flavour:

'Thank you so much for a fantastic week – it was BRILLIANT! It was such a wonderfully nurturing POSITIVE environment, a real breath of fresh air. The juices were delicious and your talks were soooo enjoyable and fun.' **Hayley**

'I loved every minute – the talks, the physical activity, the beautiful walks to the private beach, team-games (I haven't played like that since my school days!) the delicious juices and healthy food, the inspirational films, documentaries and audio, and especially the visualization Grand Design process on the last two days. You organized the week extremely well – it's difficult to imagine how you could have improved on it.' **Julie**